When Poor Was Healthy

How a Healthy Lifestyle Can Prevent and Reverse Chronic Diseases

By Getty Israel, MPH

ISBN 978-0-615-87761-7

Cover image © Mike Monahan | Dreamstime.com
Book and cover design: Darlene and Dan Swanson • www.van-garde.com

Disclaimer:

The information provided in this book is intended for health educational purposes only, not to replace the medical advice of your health care provider. The publisher and author specifically disclaim any liability, loss or risk- personal or otherwise- that is incurred as a consequence—directly or indirectly—of the use and application of any of the contents of this book. The personal stories shared in this book are personal to the users and may not reflect the results you will have if you follow the information provided in this book.

To my family and community.

A special appreciation to the following people for their contributions:

Anna Green, Fred Barnes, Rhonda Burton, Tawanna Chapman, Linda Green, Lucinda Green, Gary Griffin, Dr. Frances Henderson, Linda Jackson, Johnny Minninger, Susan Stonecypher, Tarah Mannery, Andrew Thomas, Don and Anne Turner, Stacy Turner, Lisa Whittington, and Don Williams.

Contents

PART I

Poverty or Poor Behavior

CHAPTER 1

Lessons from My Childhood

"I may be poor, but I've got my health; if you don't have good health, all the money in the world won't matter." That's what I recall my parents saying to us when I was growing up in rural Mississippi.

My childhood community was composed primarily of uninsured working poor people. In spite of poverty, we managed to live vibrant and healthy lives. Being over-weight was uncommon, and it primarily occurred among the elderly who had become sedentary. Obese children were so rare that they were considered an anomaly. Essentially, we were thin and healthier than Mississippians are today because we consistently lived an overall healthier lifestyle.

A large amount of our foods was derived from the ubiquitous family vegetable gardens and the wide variety of fruits, sugar cane, and pecans that grew wild throughout our community. Families ate a primarily fresh plant based diet that was supplemented with locally raised chicken and pork and fresh fish. Rich foods, which are now commonplace, were reserved for holidays and social events.

Processed foods were derived from fresh fruits that we gathered and preserved in canning jars. The entire family shared ice cream and cookies while watching a television program. We drank homemade lemonade and iced tea but only during dinner. Meats were home cooked but rarely fried, grilled, or barbequed. Our nearly wholesome diet was supplemented with plenty of physical activity.

We burned significantly more calories than we consumed through our daily activities. The young and old got plenty of exercise and vitamin D from the sun as we spent a considerable amount of time outdoors, often running barefoot from sunrise to sunset. When we were not in school or performing chores, we rode our bikes or walked. I recall us walking regularly for miles to visit neighbors and family. In fact, it was common for families to go for evening walks after dinner.

Essentially, we were robust as our diet and lifestyle made it nearly impossible for us to become overweight, obese, or sick. We only visited the doctor for annual school physical exams and immunizations, of which we received about 6. In contrast, children presently receive 49 doses of 14 vaccines before the age of six. Yet, ear infections, viral infections, and other common childhood illnesses were rare in my neighborhood.

The Tree

My mother, who has reared 7 children, believes that our family's way of life laid the foundation for good health, and the culture maintained it:

> For one thing, we lived off the land and raised or gathered nearly all of our foods. We rarely bought food from a supermarket. So, if you were going to eat, somebody had to produce it and cook it. When I did domestic work I would get up early and cook the day's meals before leaving for work or I would return early enough to cook dinner before my children returned home from school. I cooked plenty of vegetables and beans, and there was no junk food. The milk was fresh and came directly from the cattle in the pasture. It was healthier, and it lasted longer than milk sold in stores today. We used to drink rain water that fell in the cistern, but now there is too much pollution. The family would gather and preserve wild blackberries,

> figs, plums, and muscadines that are now nearly impossible to find because lumber companies have destroyed a lot of the natural habitat. I made sure my children took a tablespoon of cod liver oil every day; it's good for the digestive system and helps prevent colds. And, we walked nearly everywhere. Children played outside every day, even when it was cold. There was very little television time and only one television in the home.

Except the Human Feet

My childhood community has been supplanted by one that is sedentary and unhealthy. Vegetable gardens, home cooked meals, walking and bicycling have been replaced by junk foods, soft drinks, SUVs and ATVs and restaurants, especially fast food chains. Now, the young and old suffer and die of the same preventable and reversible diseases for which they receive countless drug medications, invasive therapies, and recurring hospitalizations.

Heart disease, cancer, and diabetic-induced amputations have become so prevalent that it is no longer shocking when my mother calls to inform me that another neighbor, childhood friend, or relative has prematurely died or lost her or his quality of life. Obesity, which is a leading cause of these diseases, is so pervasive that individuals of healthy weight are rare.

My mother believes that the community's poor health is the result of its modern lifestyle:

> Today, parents and children alike are overweight and unhealthy because they eat too much fast food and drink too many soft drinks. They also watch too much TV. The road is filled with all kinds of vehicles except the human feet. Parents don't cook much in today's world because

> their work schedules and long travel to work don't allow it. When my children were young, parents had less education, money, and job opportunities, but our families were much healthier. I guess you could say it was a trade off, but I'm not sure it was worth it.

Moving Beyond Poverty

Mississippi persists in leading the southern region and the nation in having the worst health. It has the highest rates of infant and adult mortality, which is nearly 30 percent higher than the U.S. mortality rate.[1-2] According to many public health experts, poverty is the leading cause of Mississippi's dire health problems.

It seems Mississippi has been a poor state forever, but its citizens have not always experienced such high rates of obesity and preventable chronic diseases. Poverty is and will likely remain an important factor in the State's health. But, is poverty the dominant cause of chronic diseases among most Mississippians?

In addition to income and education, lifestyle is a strong predictor, maybe stronger, of one's health. There are shared behaviors among groups of all socio-economic statuses that place them at risk of developing preventable chronic diseases such as hypertension, high blood cholesterol, diabetes mellitus, cardiovascular disease, and cancer. These behaviors have not always been dominant among Mississippians as many in this predominant rural state had childhood experiences similar to those in my community.

Many of us have known poverty up close and personal, but it has not prevented us from making healthy choices, such as eating healthy, exercising, and refraining from tobacco and alcohol use. Despite not having medical insurance, we have successfully prevented chronic and infectious diseases through our lifestyles.

Presently, there is a growing trend among Mississippians- and Americans- to re-embrace healthy living, and fortunately, local governments, employers, and retailers are responding. They are making major changes to meet the demands of health conscious people. In this book, you will meet some who are living proof that a healthy lifestyle can prevent and reverse chronic diseases.

This book also provides a wealth of research findings to prove the therapeutic benefits of healthy living. Although this book is written with Mississippians in mind, its message is applicable to the rest of the nation, especially those individuals who reside in states that have very similar public health challenges.

Overall, despite your level of education, income, race or genetic predisposition, there are modest changes you can begin making now to substantially improve your health. Remember, the ability to prevent and reverse most chronic diseases is within your control, not your physician, pharmacist, or insurer. The most powerful therapy on the face of the Earth is not drug medications, dietary supplements, or invasive medical procedures; rather, it is a healthy lifestyle.

We are the cure.

Chapter 2

Modern Lifestyles and Old-fashioned Diseases

Over the past 50 years, the American lifestyle has undergone modern changes that have led to an explosion in obesity and obesity-related chronic diseases. This chapter examines some of those changes: a dramatic decrease in home cooked meals and a corresponding increase in the over consumption of ultra processed foods, sweetened beverages, alcohol, and tobacco.

The Processed Food Explosion

Ironically, to a large degree, U.S. agricultural policies are responsible for the excessive availability of many unhealthy foods, beverages, and tobacco. Moreover, the U.S. federal farm subsidy program contradicts and weakens U.S. public health policies. It spends billions of public dollars to subsidize the production of unhealthy foods, beverages, and tobacco while encouraging Americans to eat healthy and stop using tobacco, the most lethal commodity in the world.

The federal farm subsidy program was established during the Great Depression to provide a safety net for family farms to maintain the nation's food supply. Like most public programs, there were negative unintended consequences, such as corporate farms receiving huge subsidies and the subsequent abundance of cheap, unhealthy foods and drinks.

Over the years, large profitable farmers of *commodity crops* have received the bulk of U.S. subsidies to grow crops that feed livestock or are used as sweeteners or other additives. For instance, merely 3.8 percent of farmers account for 75 percent of the $292.5 billion in subsidies; 62 percent of farmers received no subsidies, according to the Environmental Working Group.(3)

Of the $292.5 billion spent to subsidize U.S. commodity crops from 1995 to 2012, U.S. corn growers received $84.4 billion, and dairy and beef growers, $5.3 billion and $4 billion, respectively. The tobacco industry, ranked 14th on the subsidy list, received $1.5 billion. During that same period, apple growers, ranked 19th, received merely $261,540,987.(4)

Growers of other fruits, vegetables, and tree nuts received no subsidies at all because they are defined as *specialty crops.* Furthermore, farmers who participate in the U.S. subsidy program are prohibited from growing vegetables and fruits on the land for which they receive huge subsidies. Undoubtedly, this policy is responsible for the high retail costs of fresh fruits and vegetables. And, it has led to the mass production of ultra-processed foods and beverages that are cheap, inexpensive, ubiquitous, and overly consumed.(5)

The U.S. subsidy food program and modern lifestyle shifts have completely changed what, when, and how often Americans eat. For instance, many Americans have replaced freshly prepared home cooked meals with ultra-processed foods. These cheap foods have little nutritional value and are "formulated to be sensually appealing, hyper-palatable, and habit-forming, by the use of sophisticated mixtures of cosmetic and other additives, and state-of-the-craft packaging and marketing," according to Dr. Carlos Monteiro, Professor of Nutrition and Public Health at the University of Sao Paulo, Brazil.(6)

Dr. Monteiro has argued that wholesome traditional meals once shared by the entire family have been replaced by degraded and cheap ultra-processed foods that are designed by transnational food corporations to meet the time but not nutritional demands of busy workers, especially mothers, who no longer have time to prepare and cook meals. Subsequently, the dramatic rise in the consumption of ultra-processed foods and beverages are the main dietary cause of the world's obesity rates and obesity related chronic diseases.[(7)]

Additionally, Americans have increased the number of meals they eat in restaurants. In 1955, the restaurant industry earned 25 percent of the total amount Americans spent on food. That amount has increased to nearly 50 percent. About 66 percent of adults have reported that "their favorite restaurant foods provide flavor and taste sensations which cannot easily be duplicated in their home kitchen," according to the National Restaurant Association. Those sentiments translated into $632 billion ($1.7 billion avg/per day) Americans spent at restaurants in 2012, and sales were projected to reach $660.5 billion in 2013. Of those amounts, Mississippians spent $3.3 billion and an estimated $3.4 billion in 2012 and 2013, respectively.[(8)]

Fast-Food Industry

A considerable portion of those sales took place at fast food restaurants. Sales increased from $6 billion in 1970[(9)] to $16.1 billion in 1975[(10)] and to $117 billion in 2009. Presently, McDonalds and Subway lead the market in sales with $35.6 million and $12.1 million, respectively.[(11)]

Although both are fast-food restaurants, Subway promotes its menu as healthy. According to Yale University's Rudd Center for Food Policy and Obesity, Subway and Taco Bell do have a higher "overall nutritional quality of food items and reasonable median calories" than their competitors.[(12)] On the other hand, many of Subway's sandwiches contain high levels of sodium, which brings into question the American Heart Association's endorsement of some Subway meals as *"heart healthy"*.

Subway is a national sponsor of the American Heart Association's *My Heart. My Life.* And it is the first fast-food restaurant to receive the organization's *heart check for healthy meals.*[(13-14)] According to the American Heart Association, "these meals meet the Heart-Check's nutritional criteria for levels of sodium, calories, cholesterol, saturated fat, and trans-fats,[15] but excluding the *veggie lite* sandwich, all of the heart healthy dry meals are high in sodium.

Most of the meals exceed 800 mg. For that reason, customers would need to be careful when choosing other meals and snacks during the day to prevent exceeding the recommended daily 2400mg of sodium. In addition, the American Heart Association does not account for the possibility that consumers add generous amounts of mayonaise, cheese, and/or pickles when ordering the dry sandwiches.

University of California researchers reported Subway's sandwiches were high in sodium.[16] The study involved adolescents who consumed meals that contained three times the amount of sodium recommended by the Institute of Medicine. The amount of sodium averaged 2,149 mg and 1,829 mg for Subway and McDonald's, respectively.

Subway promotes its menu as being fresh, but many of its items contain artificial ingredients, fillers, bulking agents, processing aids, and preservatives, such as sodium nitrate, sodium benzoate, and sodium erythorbate, among others.[17] Furthermore, its foods are low in fiber, and its desserts are high in sugar and contain artificial flavors.[18] The reality is it too sells ultra processed foods.

Fast-Food Accessibility

Since the mid-1970s, the prevalence of obesity has increased by 50 percent, and obesity-induced diseases like diabetes and heart disease have risen concurrently.[19] During the same period, the number of fast-food restaurants more than doubled.[20]

A considerable number of studies have reported a strong correlation between fast-food consumption and obesity rates among urban and/or rural populations.[21-27] Fast-food restaurants are often situated and promoted within low income communities. Billboards that promote fast-food are less prominent in upper income areas regardless of the population's dominant race.[28] Fast-food restaurants tend to be more widely available in low income and/or predominantly Black communities.[29-30] For example, the largest county in Mississippi is Hinds County, which is predominantly Black. It has a median annual household income of $39,290.[31]

Hinds County has far more fast-food restaurants compared with its two neighbors, Madison County and Rankin County. Both counties are primarily comprised of Whites and have significantly larger annual household incomes.

An argument could be made that the number of fast-food restaurants is influenced by population size, but within each county there are notably more fast-food restaurants situated within predominantly Black neighborhoods. The high availability of fast-food restaurants within these neighborhoods is associated with greater caloric intake among Black adults under the age of 55, mainly among young adults and of all income levels.[32]

A similar trend exists in other predominantly Black neighborhoods, such as New Orleans, Louisiana where predominantly Black neighborhoods have over 2.5 fast-food restaurants per square mile compared with 1.5 fast-food establishments in predominantly White neighborhoods, according to Tulane University researchers.[33] The adverse health effects caused by an over consumption of fast-foods has been compounded by a substantial increase in the consumption of sweetened (sugar and high fructose corn syrup) foods and especially beverages.

High Fructose Corn Syrup

The U.S. is the world's largest consumer of sweeteners.[34] Approximately 50 percent of added sweeteners in the typical American diet are derived from sports and energy drinks, coffee beverages, fruit juices, sweet tea, and soft drinks.

Per capita soft drink consumption has increased by nearly 500 percent over the past 50 years.[35] In 1942, the U.S. soft drink industry produced about 60 twelve ounce servings per person of carbonated soft drinks. By 2005 that figure had increased nearly 10-fold.

The size of the soft drink container has soared as well. The typical soft drink container size was 6 ½ oz during the 1950s, but by 2000, it had grown to 24 oz.[36] As the container size has increased so has consumption of the ubiquitous high fructose corn syrup (HFCS) that accounts for 52 percent of sweeteners used in the U.S.[37]

Most Americans are exposed to HFCS through soft drinks as it is the exclusive sweetener used by the industry. The beverage industry accounts for over 90 percent of total domestic deliveries of HFCS. About 10 teaspoons of HFCS are added to a 12 oz can and 17 teaspoons to a 20 oz bottle.

In the U.S., HFCS consumption increased by more than 1000 percent between 1970 and 1990.[38] Eventually it replaced sugar as the number 1 sweetener during the mid 2000s. During this period, over 500 million bushels of corn was used to produce HFCS through a process called "corn wet milling".[39]

As stated earlier, corn is the number 1 subsidized crop in the U.S., which explains why HFCS is substantially less expensive than sugar. Because HFCS is cheaper, and more flexible and sweeter, it has become very popular within the food and beverage industries: processed foods, cereal and bakery producers, multiple-use food manufacturers, dairy, and the confectionery industry.[40]

It is used as an ingredient in many processed foods and beverages; consequently, the typical American consumer is likely to come in contact with it at some point during the day. Like table sugar, it too is associated with obesity, but some public health experts have shown that it has a more detrimental effect.

Princeton University researchers investigated the role of HFCS on bodyweight and triglycerides in male and female rats and found that rats that consumed a HFCS-sweetened diet gained significantly more weight and experienced higher triglycerides compared with those that received a diet sweetened with table sugar. The female rats within the HFCS group experienced abdominal obesity and higher levels of triglycerides.[41] Another animal study conducted by West Virginia University scientists found that

HFCS caused a faster gain in weight and a longer reproductive cycle.[42]

These findings suggest that individuals who consume beverages and foods sweetened with HFCS may have a greater risk of gaining more weigh. On the other hand, there is the possibility that HFCS poses a greater health risk than sugar because of its pervasiveness in most ultra-processed foods and beverages, especially soft drinks.[43]

Many overweight and obese individuals drink large amounts of sweetened beverages from which they derive a considerable percentage of their daily calories. For example, one study showed that nearly 11 percent of overweight adults consumed more than 450 calories per day from sweetened drinks.[44] In another study that involved children, for each additional serving of sweetened beverages consumed, they experienced a significant risk of becoming obese.[45] Obesity can cause metabolic syndrome, which leads to other chronic conditions such as type 2 diabetes, hypertension, gout, and cardiovascular disease.

Sweetened Beverages and Health

Metabolic Syndrome

Metabolic syndrome, also known as cardio-metabolic syndrome, is defined as a person having 3 or more of the following conditions:

- waist circumference ≥35 inches for women or ≥40 inches for men;
- fasting blood sugar ≥100 mg/dL or treatment with oral hypoglycemic agents or insulin;
- blood pressure ≥135/85 mm Hg or treatment for hypertension;
- serum triglycerides ≥150 mg/dL or
- HDL <40 mg/dL in men or <50 mg/dL in women.

Consuming soft drinks has been shown to rapidly raise blood glucose and insulin levels,[46] which increases the risk of developing metabolic syndrome. Metabolic syndrome substantially increases the risk of individuals developing other conditions such as type 2 diabetes.

Type 2 diabetes

There is a strong association between the regular consumption (1-2 servings per day) of sweetened beverages and the risk of developing type 2 diabetes.[47] However, drinking caffeinated coffee and tea is associated with a lower risk among men and women, respectively.[48] Merely replacing 1 serving of sweetened beverage with 1 cup of coffee may substantially lower the risk of diabetes among men.[49] Women who decrease their daily consumption of sweetened beverages may reduce their risk of gaining weight and subsequently developing type 2 diabetes.[50]

The high consumption of sweetened beverages is likely a major factor in the high rates of obesity, metabolic syndrome, and diabetes among Blacks. Among all age groups, Blacks have the highest consumption rates of sweetened beverages.[51] Black women have an average daily amount of calories from sweetened beverages that is double that of White females.[52] They also have the highest prevalence of type 2 diabetes.[53]

According to a Boston University study, Black women who drank 2 or more sweetened beverages soft drinks and fruit beverages per day experienced an average 27.5 percent increase in type 2 diabetes.[54] A high consumption of sweetened beverages may be a contributing factor in the very high rates of hypertension among Black women, who happen to develop it at an earlier age than other groups.[55]

Hypertension

There is a strong relationship between regular consumption of sweetened beverages, serum uric acid levels, and hypertension among various groups of adolescents and adults.[56-57] HFCS and sugar are made up of glucose and fructose. Fructose is reported to acutely decrease urinary sodium excretion, thereby potentially raising systemic blood pressure in young healthy individuals.[58] It is absorbed and digested differently than glucose. Fructose is absorbed farther down the intestine, and it is primarily metabolized in the liver [59-60] where it produces uric acid.[61]

Serum uric acid is another important risk factor for developing hypertension[62-66] and cardio-metabolic syndrome among children and adolescents,[67] the largest consumers of sweetened beverages. Teens who consume high levels of sweetened beverages may experience increased levels of serum uric acid and systolic blood pressure.[68] Black youth, who tend to have higher levels of systolic blood pressure[69] and the highest consumption of soft drinks, have a greater risk of developing hypertension.[70] Developing high levels of serum uric acid during childhood is strongly associated with adult hypertension among adolescents of both genders.[71]

Gout

Excessive uric acid is linked to gout,[72] a form of arthritis, as well. In addition to excessive alcohol use, gout may be caused by regular consumption of sweetened beverages among women[73] and men.[74] Men who drank 2 or more servings of soft drinks per day were found to have an 85 percent higher risk of developing gout compared with men who consumed less than 1 serving per month.[75]

Gout occurs more often in men, but women are also at risk, particularly those who consume excessive amounts of fructose. A study by researchers at Boston University showed that as women increased their consumption of soda and orange juice, their risk of developing gout also increased.[76]

Cardiovascular Disease

Men and women who regularly consume sweetened beverages may have an increased risk of developing cardiovascular disease. Women who drank 2 or more soft drinks, punches, or fruit drinks were significantly more likely to develop coronary heart disease than those women who consumed less than 1 beverage.[77] Men who regularly drank sweetened beverages experienced a 19% increased risk of developing coronary heart disease.[78]

Frequent intake of sweetened beverages may heighten the risk of a stroke. Women who regularly drank sweetened soda were found to have a higher risk of ischemic stroke, whereas those who consumed diet soda experienced a higher risk of hemorrhagic stroke. In contrast, coffee drinkers experienced a lower risk of stroke.[79]

Bone Fractures

Regular consumption of sweetened beverages has a negative effect on bones, especially among females. Studies have reported an increased risk of bone fractures among adolescent girls and women, but not boys and men. Reports have shown that older women who frequently drank cola experienced significantly lower bone mineral density in the hip areas.[80]

Adolescent girls who frequently consumed cola beverages experienced low bone mineral accumulation during peak bone mass accrual,[81] an increased risk of wrist and forearm fractures,[82] and bone fractures. The negative effects on bones mostly occurred in physically active girls but not boys.[83] Carbonated soft drinks have been implicated in reducing bone mineral density at the heel in girls but not boys.[84]

Overall, the high intake of sweetened beverages is a major contributor to obesity, obesity-induced chronic conditions, and bone fractures. Reducing consumption levels of these types of beverages would likely cause a considerable decline in obesity rates, particularly abdominal obesity, and related diseases. To this end, public health experts have pushed for policies to reduce sweetened beverage consumption rates among children and adolescents. Many school administrations have responded by restricting the sale of sweetened beverages on campus, but such efforts are weakened by parents who persist in making these drinks available in the home and at fast-food restaurants.

Alcohol

Excessive alcohol consumption is the third leading preventable cause of chronic disease, injury, and death in the U.S.[85] Persistent and extreme alcohol consumption can lead to fatty liver, alcoholic hepatitis, alcoholic cirrhosis, and cancer.[86]

The state of Mississippi is a good example of the deleterious effects of excessive alcohol use. Although current alcohol consumption in Mississippi is among the lowest in the nation, its sales of alcoholic beverages have increased considerably over the past 50 years. From 1967 to 2011, the state experienced a 93 percent increase in net proceeds from alcohol sales within its 48 wet counties.[87]

Mississippi is one of 18 Control states, which means it directly manages the sale of alcoholic beverages at the wholesale level. Its 27.5 percent markup on alcoholic beverages yields nearly $50 million in annual net proceeds, and it collects about $42.4 million in taxes and fees associated with regulating alcohol. On the other hand, it incurs $2.1 million annually in medical related costs caused by excessive alcohol use.[88] This figure does not include the high costs associated with loss of life, quality of life, and productivity.

The State's steady climb in alcohol sales parallels the rise in alcohol related diseases and deaths in the state. Among Mississippians, alcohol is responsible for 31 percent and 66 percent of chronic and acute causes of death, respectively. Homicides and suicides account for 19 percent and 12 percent, respectively, of acute deaths associated with alcohol.[89]

Furthermore, alcohol is a leading cause of traffic related mortalities, accounting for 37 percent in the state.[90] In addition to impairing the driver, it increases the probability that the driver and occupants will not wear a seatbelt, primarily at night.

Nationally, alcohol impaired drivers make up more than two-thirds of drivers killed at night. Only 26 percent of those drivers wear seatbelts, according to a report from the National Highway Traffic Safety Administration.[91] Alcohol was likely a contributing factor in the deaths of nearly

50 percent of Mississippi occupants who were not restrained during vehicular mortalities.[92]

Tobacco

Tobacco remains the leading cause of preventable disease and death in the nation. It is associated with a wide variety of chronic diseases such as cardiovascular disease and various forms of cancer. Yet, Americans smoke 350 billion cigarettes annually, accounting for more than 440,000 deaths in the U. S.

Tobacco use persists in being a serious public health problem in Mississippi, which has the 5th highest percentage of smokers in the nation,[93] and the 2nd highest percentage of adults who consume smokeless tobacco.[94]

Approximately 4700 Mississippians die each year from smoking, and 192,000 children are exposed to secondhand smoke.[95] The state has the 2nd highest death rate of lung and bronchus cancer. The disease costs Mississippi $662 million annually for medical care,[96] which is exceedingly greater than the $263 million it earns in tobacco revenue.

For the most part, tobacco consumption, excessive alcohol use, diets primarily comprised of ultra processed foods and sweetened beverages and a sedentary lifestyle have all contributed substantially to the prevalence of obesity and chronic conditions that have exploded over the past decades in Mississippi and the nation. Moreover, even though this modern unhealthy lifestyle appears to be widespread among the poor, it is not exclusive as a considerable number of middle and upper income people also practice similar unhealthy lifestyles that lead to chronic diseases and premature deaths.

Nonetheless, data consistently show that when people adopt healthy behaviors their health improves. Therefore the risk of developing or dying of a chronic disease can be substantially reduced among all groups despite their race and/or socio-economic status.

Chapter 3

Race and Health Disparities

Blacks are consistently reported to experience the worst health in the U. S. Being Black has quietly become defined as a *risk factor* for developing most preventable diseases: cardiovascular disease, type 2 diabetes, hypertension, renal disease, common cancers, and sexually transmitted diseases.

A risk factor is something that increases a person's likelihood of developing or dying of a disease or injury. Some factors, e.g. race, age, are uncontrollable whereas others, e.g. personal behavior, are controllable. When controllable risk factors are changed or eliminated the disease, injury, or subsequent death can be prevented or delayed. Controllable risk factors include: diet, tobacco exposure, excessive alcohol use, physical inactivity, and obesity.

In the case of Blacks, public health experts would have us believe that race and/or poverty are chiefly responsible for their poor health. This was certainly the case when Blacks experienced open, legal, and institutionalized racism, hence, denied economical opportunities, sanitary living conditions, and medical care, among others.

A Normal Human Being

W.E.B. DuBois tackled the role of poverty Black's health in his 1906 article, the *Health and Physique of the Negro American*. The document was part of the proceedings of the Eleventh Conference for the Study of the Negro

Problem in Atlanta, GA. DuBois convincingly argued that the high mortality rates of Northern Blacks- which were lower than that of Southern Blacks- were caused not by racial inferiority or vulnerability to the cold climate but social conditions rooted in poverty. He wrote:

> The undeniable fact is, then, that in certain diseases the Negroes have a much higher rate than the whites, and especially in consumption [tuberculosis], pneumonia and infantile diseases. The question is: Is this racial? Mr. Hoffman would lead us to say yes, and to infer that it means that Negroes are inherently inferior in physique to whites... With the improved sanitary condition, improved education and better economic opportunities, the mortality of the race may and probably will steadily decrease until it becomes normal... The Conference does not find any adequate scientific warrant for the assumption that the Negro race is inferior to other races in physical build or vitality. The present differences in mortality seem to be sufficiently explained by conditions of life; and physical measurements prove the Negro a normal human being capable of average human accomplishments.

Nearly eight decades after the Atlanta Conference, Margaret Heckler, Secretary of Health and Human Services, released the *Report of the Secretary's Task Force on Black and Minority Health.* She examined critical differences in the quality of health between Whites and Blacks. Subsequently, federal laws were passed. Federal initiatives, funding, and offices were created to address health disparities among Blacks. Some include: the Office on Research of Minority Health, the National Center on Minority Health and Health Disparities, the Excellence Centers to Eliminate Ethnic/Racial Disparities, the Office of Minority Health, and the National Institute on Minority Health and Health Disparities, among others.

Despite public and private sector efforts and the substantial social, political, educational, and economical gains of the Civil Rights era and beyond, Blacks persist in having the worse health in the nation. This is especially evident in southern states, which have higher proportions of Black residents than the rest of the nation, excluding New York and California. Although poverty remains a barrier, it does not appear to be the dominant underlying cause of morbidity and mortality among most present-day Blacks.

The poverty factor is highly questionable when considering the $695.6 billion overall combined household income of Blacks and the $87 billion in annual buying power of affluent Blacks,(97) who often experience similar health issues as Blacks and Whites with lower income.

Presently, Blacks experience cardiovascular disease and cancer mortality rates higher than they did during the 50's and 60's. For instance, in 1950, the overall heart disease mortality rate of Blacks was nearly the same as Whites. By 1960, it was significantly lower than that of Whites, but by 1970 it had risen sharply among Blacks. Within 30 years, it had increased 30 percent higher than that of Whites. The same trend is true of Blacks' overall cancer mortality rate, which was significantly lower than that of Whites in 1950, but it jumped 40 percent higher 50 years later.(98)

Currently, Blacks of every income level have a higher coronary heart disease mortality rate than that of Whites. For example, compared with low and middle income White women, Black women of the same income levels experience heart disease mortality rates 65 percent and 50 percent higher, respectively.(99)

Furthermore, cardiovascular disease was not the number 1 killer of Blacks in 1906, according to DuBois. In fact, he identified consumption (tuberculosis), cholera infantum (gastroenteritis), and infantile marasmus (a wasting disease) as the leading causes of mortality among Blacks. These diseases were associated with malnutrition, deplorable sanitary conditions, and lack of quality medical care.

In contrast, today, unhealthy lifestyles are primarily responsible for the high rates of infant mortality and chronic diseases. At present, Blacks in general have greater resources, better living conditions, and greater access to medical care. Yet, even when socio-economic factors are equal among Blacks and Whites, Blacks persist in having the worse outcomes. A closer examination reveals tobacco use and obesity at the center of health disparities among Blacks. Therefore, unhealthy behaviors, e.g. physical inactivity, diet and smoking, are probably chiefly responsible for the disproportionately high rates of diseases Blacks experience.

For instance, tobacco use is especially prevalent among Black men as they continue to experience higher rates of tobacco consumption and related diseases than other groups. High tobacco use was not always common among Black men. From 1901 to 1940, for example, Black men had a lower smoking rate than that of White men, but they began to smoke significantly more during the latter part of the century.(100) Excluding 2004, their smoking rates have continued to outpace that of White males each year.(101)

During the mid-50s, studies began to link tobacco with chronic diseases. White males stopped smoking in huge numbers, but smoking rates among Black males did not begin to decline until a decade or so later when they were much older than White males.(102) Anti-smoking messages did not appear on television until the late 1960s, which may have contributed to the difference in smoking cessation rates among Black and White males. Anti-smoking messages also were being countered by the advent of filtered cigarettes, and the abundance of menthol cigarette advertising campaigns that appeared primarily in Black publications and in Black communities.

Overall, persistent smoking, an unhealthy diet, low physical activity levels, and a late diagnosis are more likely the underlying causes of Black men experiencing the highest mortality rates of heart disease and lung cancer in the nation. Additionally, obesity, the 2nd leading cause of chronic diseases and mortality in the U.S.,(103) substantially affects the health of Black men and women of all income levels.

Blacks have the highest obesity rates in the nation. More than 30 percent of Blacks, who reside in over 41 states, are obese or overweight. In contrast, 30 percent of overweight or obese Whites reside in only four states.[(104)] In Mississippi, which has the 3rd highest rate of physical inactivity, Blacks have an obesity rate of 43 percent.

Obesity has extreme adverse effects on the health of Black women, who happen to have the highest obesity rates in every state in which they reside, except for Maine, Iowa, Minnesota, New Mexico, Arizona, and Connecticut, where Mexican women are the most obese.[(105)]

Approximately 82 percent of Black women and 75 percent of Mexican women are overweight or obese.[(106)] Over half of Black women who are age 20 or older are obese.[(107)] By the age of 39, the average body mass index (BMI) of Black women is greater than 30 kg/m^2, the cut-off point for obesity. What's more, obesity is a strong indicator of reproductive health problems.

Maternal obesity increases the risk of poor birthing outcomes, which probably explains why Black women have the nation's highest infant mortality rates every year. Black women are approximately 60 percent more likely than White women to experience premature births that can lead to infant mortality. Black babies are about 230 percent more likely than White babies to die before their first birthday.[(108)]

Infant mortality is associated with obesity-induced hypertension and type 2 diabetes, pre-existing conditions Black women are more likely to have when they become pregnant or during pregnancy. Obese women are more likely to have pregnancy-induced gestational diabetes, venous thromboembolism (the formation of a blood clot in a deep vein), overweight newborns, and miscarriages during the latter half of their pregnancies and a higher incidence of wound infections related to cesarean section births,[(109)] of which Black women have the highest rate (36 percent).[(110)] Additionally, maternal obesity increases the risk of babies having a range of structural abnormalities[(111)] and a substantial increase of central nervous system birth defects.[(112)]

Reproductive health should improve as a woman's income and/or education increases, but unlike White women, Black women's birthing outcomes do not improve with higher education or income. Interestingly, Black women with undergraduate and graduate level education have a higher infant mortality rate than that of White women who have not completed high school.(113)

Furthermore, the suggestion that obesity is an exclusive problem among all poor people is questionable as most obese adults are not low-income, according to one study.(114) The study found that the influence of income on obesity varied by race, ethnicity, and gender. At the highest income level, Whites, especially White women, had notably lower obesity rates than Blacks and Mexicans. White women were significantly less likely to be obese as their income levels increased. Black women and Mexican women experienced insignificant lower obesity rates at higher income levels(115)

Among White men, obesity was comparable at all income levels. Surprisingly, Black men and Mexican men who had incomes below 130 percent of the poverty level were **significantly less likely** to be obese compared with Black and Mexican men who possessed higher incomes.(116)

Generally, men and women who were college graduates had a lower obesity rate than those who were not. College educated White men and women had the lowest obesity rates followed by Mexican men and women. College educated Black men and women had the highest obesity rates.

Black female college graduates also have been found to have an obesity rate about two times that of White women and Mexican women. (117) Among White women and Mexican women, those with college degrees were **significantly less likely** to be obese than women who had less than a high school degree. However, a college education did not translate into lower obesity rates among Black women.

Higher education and income are expected to improve one's health. This is typically the case among Whites as they tend to have lower rates of obesity and an overall greater health status than Whites with less education and income. For some reason, an increase in socio-economic status does not translate into good health among Blacks, particularly Black women.

College educated, higher earning Blacks often have obesity and chronic disease rates similar to those of Blacks with less education and income. Middle and upper income Blacks have greater access to health information and primary medical care, but they often practice similar unhealthy behaviors as lower income Blacks, such as physical inactivity and unhealthy diets. The evidence convincingly shows that unhealthy lifestyles, which lead to obesity, are primarily responsible for the poor health of most Blacks. Yet, when Blacks, of all income levels, make healthy lifestyle changes they improve their health and extend their lives.

Half the battle in reducing obesity and subsequent health disparities among Blacks, particularly Black women, is convincing them that they have a weight problem. Studies have found that an individual's inability to recognize that she is clinically overweight is strongly linked to that person's probability of becoming obese.[(118-119)]

Racially diverse studies on perception and weight have found that Black females do not recognize they are overweight or obese. A study reported that overweight Black women within the reproductive age group were more likely to perceive themselves as normal weight.[(120)] In another study involving women between 20 and 39 years of age, twice as many overweight Black women saw themselves as being normal weight. Other studies have drawn similar conclusions about Black women and Black female adolescents.[(121-122)]

Black women have reported the following reasons why some do not attempt to lose weight: a desire not to be thin, family members' satisfaction with their weight, dislike of physical activity because of perspiration and appearance, program access barriers, and difficulties with clothing.[(123)] Additionally, some Black women believe the BMI does not provide an accurate measurement of their body weight and frame. They also face less social pressure to lose weight, and they often appear to be satisfied with their higher body weight.

Genetic Predisposition:

Why are Blacks predisposed to high rates of chronic diseases? Being genetically predisposed to a disease indicates the existence of an inherent flaw, which is not the case for the majority of Blacks. However, high rates of obesity and/or smoking are common risk factors among most Black adults. For instance, Blacks have the highest rates of hypertension, which makes them susceptible to disproportionately high rates of heart disease. On the other hand, they also have the highest rates of obesity, and one of the highest rates of cigarette smoking, which predisposes them to disproportionately higher rates of hypertension and heart disease.

So, reducing obesity and smoking rates among Blacks should be the primary goal of any racially based health disparity program. In Mississippi, racial health disparities are often cited as justification to fund new initiatives. Although such funding generously benefits nonprofit public health organizations, disparities persist among Blacks. This is primarily because program administrators either ignore or marginalize the underlying behavioral issues that negatively influence Blacks' health. It is not surprising that these initiatives rarely, if ever, produce substantial improvements in their health.

Therefore, the current approach to eliminating health disparities among Blacks must drastically change to include programs that address self-perception and unhealthy behaviors. Nonprofit organizations that serve Black populations, and municipalities, states, and employers that have high proportions of Black residents and employees, respectively, must implement lifestyle change intervention programs, such as the National Diabetes Prevention Program, to target Blacks who are overweight, obese, and smoke cigarettes. In addition, Blacks must play an active role in improving their health. It's imperative that they modify or eliminate behaviors that place them at greater risk of becoming obese and developing and dying of chronic diseases.

Meanwhile, categorizing Blacks as a risk factor simply because they have disproportionately high rates of chronic diseases sends the wrong message. It discourages personal responsibility for health, undermines the ability to make healthy lifestyle choices, and diminishes the value of doing so. Moreover, it encourages medical providers to overmedicate Blacks for conditions they can prevent and reverse through practicing healthy behavior.

PART II

Moving from Medical Care to Preventive Care

...only 15 per cent of individual well-being is attributable to the pharmaceutical industry and the complex network of academic medical centers, specialist physician practices and 5,000 community-based hospitals that deliver acute care services for millions of patients. Dr. David Nash, founding Dean of the Jefferson Medical University School of Population Health.

Chapter 4

The Revolving Door

An unhealthy lifestyle, which leads to obesity and obesity related chronic diseases, is the number one reason Americans are taking drug medications, hence, over-medicated. In 2011, medically insured Americans spent $49 billion out-of-pocket for prescription drugs. Most of the spending took place in the southern region, which accounts for the nation's highest rates of obesity, heart disease, and type 2 diabetes. Southern states have the highest levels of per capita usage of prescription drugs for preventable chronic diseases.(124)

Chronic disease medication use also has spiked among children, as young as five, for treatment of type 2 diabetes, hypertension, and hyperlipidemia (high blood cholesterol).(125) Although the overall highest use in drug medications has occurred among 16 to 18 year olds, six to eleven year olds have experienced the greatest increase.

The surge in chronic disease medication therapy should be alarming because it is being used to treat diseases that are preventable and reversible through healthy lifestyle changes. Even though drug medications are FDA approved, they should not be taken lightly because they can cause serious adverse drug reactions (ADRs) that can lead to hospitalization, disability, and death.

Adverse Drug Reactions

Most recent data show that 3.2 million ADRs were reported to the FDA. Of that number, over 500,000 were deaths,[126] which are more likely to occur among individuals who are 55 and older, Black, and reside in extremely rural areas.[127] The more drugs- usually 4 or more- a person consumes, the more likely the individual will experience an ADR.

Children also have a great risk of experiencing an ADR because approximately 75 percent of drugs used by them have not been tested specifically for their use.[128] Consider that between 1995 and 2005, children 0–18 years of age made an average of 585,922 ADR related medical visits annually. The 0 to 4 year old age group accounted for 43 percent of the total, according to a report by Boston Children's Hospital. The increase in medication is driven by the current U.S. medical model and the influence of the drug industry, e.g. drug medication advertisements.

I saw it on TV

Direct-to-consumer (DTC) drug advertisements play an important role in the over use of drug medications for treating chronic diseases. DTC advertisements are designed to by-pass the medical provider and target the general public with promotional messages that tout the drug's health benefits while minimizing potentially harmful ADRs. These ads are so influential that they are banned in every nation except the U.S. and New Zealand.

In August 1997, the Food and Drug Administration (FDA) issued new guidelines for prescription drug advertising. The new guidelines allowed the industry to promote its drugs' benefits, offer a very brief summary of the major ADRs and direct viewers to the company's website for more information.[129]

The policy change has led to a huge increase in drug medication ads, some of which introduce the susceptible public to conditions they have never heard of and related new drugs. Ads touting prescription drugs have substantially grown over the last decade. In 1998, the drug industry's advertising budget was $1.2 billion,[130] and by 2009, it had increased to $4.5 billion.[131-132]

Directly marketing drugs to prospective consumers often encourages individuals to self-diagnose a purported condition and request the brand name drug featured in the advertisement. According to the FDA, 41 percent of physicians believe DTC ads cause their patients to be misinformed about the effectiveness of a drug. Also, 35 percent of physicians said they felt somewhat or very pressured to prescribe a drug when the patient requested it.(133)

Representatives of the pharmaceutical industry counter that the ads increase the public's understanding of their health and potential diseases, but researchers at the University of California have concluded DTC ads are unbalanced because they provide the public with limited information about the cause of the disease in question and adverse risk factors. The ads marginalize the role of lifestyle in healing and suggest that the drug is necessary to restore health. The "ads have limited educational value and may oversell the benefits of drugs in ways that might conflict with promoting population health," they wrote.(134)

Overall, the industry has done a masterful job of promoting chronic disease drug medications in vague simple terms while softly and quickly mentioning the potential adverse side-effects. The implication that individuals will live healthier and happier lives through drug medications increases the desire for and dependency on drugs for diseases that in most cases can be prevented or reversed through lifelong healthy living.

The Industry and Medical Education

Even though the public's understanding of drug medications is significantly influenced by DTC ads, it still relies on medical providers for the best therapy to treat a condition. However, a physician's decision is likely influenced by his association with the industry, a relationship that begins in medical school where medical students and faculty often interact with the industry.

"Financial relationships with industry are extensive in medical education," stated a Institute of Medicine (IOM) report(135) The IOM report revealed that 3rd year medical students participated in a variety of industry-sponsored social events, education events, research projects, and they received industry awards, gifts, and fellowships. It recommended that "Congress creates a national reporting program that requires pharmaceutical, medical device, and biotechnology companies to report all payments to physicians, researchers, health care institutions, professional societies, patient advocacy and disease groups and providers of medical education."(136)

To prevent conflicts of interest, some medical schools have implemented policies that forbid faculty from making promotional speeches for drug companies and accepting gifts. However, an investigative report by ProPublica revealed that these policies are ineffective because many school administrators have failed to enforce them.(137)

The federal government has taken steps to provide transparency of financial relationships between the industry, physicians, and teaching hospitals to prevent conflicts of interest and help patients make better informed health decisions. Manufacturers of drugs, biological, medical devices, and supplies must now report all payments and transfers of value to physicians and teaching hospitals and the nature of the payments to the Centers for Medicare and Medicaid Services Open Payments website.

Open Payments is a national disclosure program known as the *Physician Payment Sunshine Act,* a component of the Patient Protection Affordable Care Act. Group purchasing organizations (GPOs) are required to report investments and ownerships of physicians or their immediate family members.(138)

Nutrition and Medical Education

Although medical students and physicians are well aware of the role of drug therapies in treating chronic diseases, most do not learn much about the role of nutrition and behavior in preventing and treating chronic diseases. Consequently, the typical physician writes drug prescriptions for chronic diseases but fails to prescribe a lifestyle change plan that would address underlying factors such as diet.

"The need for nutrition counseling is pressing in light of the epidemic of chronic diseases such as hypertension, diabetes mellitus, obesity and hyperlipidemia," stated Dr. Charles B. Eaton of Brown University Medical School and the Center for Primary Care and Prevention at Memorial Hospital of Rhode Island. He found that nutrition counseling occurs in ¼ of all visits to family practice physicians and that physicians spend an average of less than a minute on nutritional therapy with their patients. Patients who suffered from acute illnesses were less likely to receive nutrition therapy.(139)

Many physicians simply do not have the training to recommend nutritional therapies to their patients. They continually rate their nutritional knowledge and skills as insufficient as most did not receive adequate nutrition education while in medical school. In 1985, the National Academy of Sciences found that nutrition education was inadequate in most U.S. medical schools.(140) The Academy recommended 25 hours of instruction for medical students, but nutrition was not taught as an exclusive course by the majority of the medical schools.

Two decades have passed since that recommendation, but nutrition education within U.S. medical schools remains inadequate.(141) In 2004, researchers at the University of North Carolina (UNC) at Chapel Hill surveyed 106 medical schools and found the overwhelming majority required some form of nutrition education. However, merely 30 percent of the schools required a separate and exclusive nutrition course. Those that required nutrition education provided an average of 23.9 contact hours. Only 41 percent of the schools met the minimum 25 hours of nutrition instruction recommended by the National Academy of Sciences.(142)

The UNC scholars revisited the issue in 2008 and found very little improvement. They reported that the majority of the 127 medical schools required some form of nutrition education, but only 25 percent of the schools required a course dedicated to nutrition. Merely 20 percent of the medical students experienced contact hours of nutrition instruction. Only 27 percent of the schools met the minimum 25 required hours recommended by the National Academy of Sciences.[143]

The Other Pills

In search of a safer alternative to drug medications and expensive doctor visits, many Americans have turned to dietary supplements. Although the ingredients (vitamins, herbs, minerals, amino acids) in dietary supplements are natural, the overwhelming majority of these products have not been proven to be safe or effective.

The Dietary Supplement Health and Education Act of 1994 (DSHEA), which governs the industry, allows the dietary supplement industry to operate under loose regulations. Unlike the pharmaceutical industry, excluding a new dietary ingredient, dietary supplement manufacturers (and distributors) are not required to obtain Food and Drug Administration (FDA) approval before marketing and selling their products.

The manufacturer is responsible for guaranteeing product safety, but the FDA does not approve product safety and efficacy before marketing. In addition, the manufacturer is responsible for evaluating its products for efficacy and content accuracy; however, it is not required by law to disclose any safety or health benefits information to the FDA or U.S. public.

This is because dietary supplements are categorized under "foods" and cannot be promoted as a "treatment, prevention, or cure for a specific disease or condition," according to the FDA. Consequently, dietary supplement manufacturers are allowed to make general health claims, structure/function claims, and nutrient content claims, but the FDA does not evaluate these claims or analyze the food content of the products.[144] If the FDA can prove that a dietary supplement is unsafe, through research and tracking adverse reactions, it can be removed from the market.

Although the public has plenty of access to adverse effects and efficacy information regarding drug medications, it is ill informed and seems less concerned about the efficacy and safety of dietary supplements. Many consumers assume that these products are safe and effective because they are believed to be natural, but natural ingredients can cause adverse effects and prove to be ineffective.

While the pharmaceutical industry promotes its drugs on TV, the dietary supplement industry has proven to be very effective in utilizing the internet to sell its products, without producing any scientific evidence to validate their claims. Often when customers request scientific evidence, sales representatives will direct them to PubMed, the federal government's database of biomedical literature, but this can be very misleading.

For instance, glucosamine sulfate is a popular dietary supplement that is commonly used to treat joint problems. There are nearly 20,000 published articles in PubMed of which only a few have shown the active ingredient to be effective. A sales representative can point to this evidence as proof that the product works, and there lies the problem. Most customers are not aware that a particular type, crystalline glucosamine sulfate, was the subject of the scientific investigations that was proved to be effective. Crystalline glucosamine sulfate is not all natural as it has some synthetic additives, but it is the only glucosamine supplement that has been shown to be effective and safe. Consequently, many customers are purchasing glucosamine related products that have never been scientifically investigated.

This is why dietary supplement manufacturers should be required to conduct clinical trials to prove the efficacy and safety of each of their products. The FDA or some other federal agency should be obligated to validate any health and content claims before they are manufactured, marketed, and placed on the shelves for susceptible customers to purchase.

Industry proponents often counter that it cannot afford the costs associated with research, and stricter regulations would be bad for business. Its $32 billion in annual sales, which are expected to reach $60 billion by 2021, screams otherwise. Furthermore, although the industry does not invest in research, it does in political influence, which has thus far managed to prevent tougher regulations.

The pharmaceutical and dietary supplement industries have powerful U.S. legislators to protect their financial interests. According to data compiled by the Center for Responsive Politics, during the 2012 election cycle, the dietary supplement industry contributed a total of $3.5 million to federal candidates and spent $2.9 million lobbying Congress.[145] In contrast, during the same election cycle, the pharmaceutical manufacturing industry contributed $21.6 million and spent $139.5 million lobbying Congress. Obviously, the latter industry is more profitable, but both have managed to convince federal legislators to protect their respective industries.

Overall, Americans are going through the revolving door from the physician's office to the pharmacy or dietary supplements store. Both groups are popping pills to treat conditions they can prevent and reverse through healthy lifestyle changes.

CHAPTER 5

Investing in Prevention

More Medical Care and Less Healing

The focus of the U.S. medical care system is not disease prevention and healing rather lifelong disease management with drug therapies, invasive therapies, and recurring hospitalizations that typically do not improve the patient's quality or length of life but often indefinitely keeps the patient in the system. According to Richard Dooling, author of *Critical Care*[146]:

> ..., expensive care is often worse care, because it snowballs into what some are calling an 'epidemic of overtreatment,' in which unnecessary procedures, tests and medications all spawn more tests, more meds (to treat the side effects of the first batch) and more follow-up scans and procedures (in stand-alone clinics owned by the same doctors prescribing the tests, scans and procedures).

One would expect that areas of the country that spend more on medical care would have a higher quality of health, but quite the opposite is true. Additional doctor visits and testing often lead to unnecessary procedures and hospitalizations that carry risks such as medical errors, adverse effects caused by medications, and infections, particularly among Medicare patients.

According to a report by Dartmouth Medical School, Medicare patients who reside in regions with higher medical spending and who receive more intensive medical care do not experience a higher rate of survival and quality of life than those patients in regions where spending is significantly lower. The patients who receive more medical care do not live longer or function better, but they have a greater risk of dying. [147-148]

The amount and type of medical care varies by region, and physicians tend to determine care based upon available medical resources, not proven therapies, severity of the illness, or the patient's preference. According to Dr. Elliot Fisher, professor of medicine at Dartmouth Medical School[149]:

> We may be wasting perhaps 30% of U.S. health care spending on medical care that does not appear to improve our health. For patients with serious illnesses (hip fracture, colorectal cancer, acute myocardial infarction) the higher intensity practice pattern was associated with a higher risk of death over time.

Most medical dollars are being used to manage chronic diseases that place huge demands on the economy. Treating people who have chronic diseases account for 83 percent of all medical care costs in the U.S., and 74 percent of private health insurance spending. Individuals who have chronic disease are more likely to have more doctor visits, hospitalizations, and to consume more drug medication.[150]

The leading chronic diseases in the U.S. and other developed countries include: hypertension, high cholesterol, cardiovascular diseases, cancer, diabetes, and arthritis. Smoking, high blood pressure and being overweight or obese are the leading causes of chronic diseases and the subsequent annual 900,000 premature deaths in the U. S. In 2008, 90 million people had at least one chronic disease, and by 2020, 157 million are expected to have at least one. Most will be treated with expensive drug therapies.

Yet, it costs less to prevent chronic diseases than to use conventional therapies. The Trust for America's Health reported that reducing the number of people who develop diabetes, hypertension, heart disease, kidney disease, and stroke by 5 percent would save the U.S. more than $19 billion in medical costs.[(151)] If the U.S. would invest a mere $10 per person/annually in community-based disease prevention programs that target diet, physical activity, and tobacco, it could save about $2.8 billion annually in medical costs in 1 to 2 years, approximately $16 billion annually within 5 years, and about $18 billion annually in 10 to 20 years.

Take Mississippi as an example. In 2012, the State incurred $719 million in medical costs directly caused by smoking and obesity. If it would invest $10 per person, it could receive a net savings of $24.3 million in 1–2 years, $150.4 million in 5 years, and $168 million within 10 – 20 years.

Shifting from Sick Care

The state of Mississippi is ranked 48th in the nation on public health spending per capita.[(152)] In 2013 and 2014, it appropriated $33.1 million and $36 million, respectively, for public health. A steady flow of external aid enters the State to help address the poor health of Mississippians.

During the previous decade, over a billion in public health funding from federal agencies and private organizations, such as the Robert Woods Johnson Foundation and the Kellogg Foundation, has poured into the State to address health disparities. Unfortunately, funding has not made a significant improvement in the health of Mississippians as high prevalence rates of obesity, cardiovascular disease, diabetes, hypertension, and common forms of cancer continue to devastate the population.

Betty Daniels, a veteran public health professional in Mississippi, believes that public health funding alone will not improve the health of Mississippians:

> Throwing dollars at the problem is not the solution. Consider the Mississippi Delta has been on the receiving end of millions of dollars from public and private sector sources for decades; yet, the overall health status of its residents remain among the lowest in the country. What then is the solution? We need a paradigm shift away from sick care to health care. This means laying aside the "sick care" practice of prescribing drugs that only treat the symptoms of disease and embracing the "health care" practice that promotes a change in the way of life that facilitates the onset of many of the chronic conditions now rampant in our culture. Health care practitioners and their patients must recognize that a healthy way of living is a far more effective treatment for obesity, type 2 diabetes, arthritis, hypertension, heart disease, etc., than a pill could ever be!

Time for a New Approach to Health

The *2014 Mississippi Health Plan* calls for hiring more physicians, nurses, physical therapists, occupational therapists, and emergency medical personnel.[153] These clinical-based professionals provide crucial medical care to patients who have already developed a chronic disease or experienced an injury that could lead to a lower quality of life or premature death.

Unfortunately, the Plan omits vital health professionals who assist the public in preventing diseases and injuries from developing or occurring through the adoption of healthy behaviors, e.g. diet, physical activity, seat belt usage, tobacco cessation, etc.

These professionals are trained to develop disease and injury prevention programs within communities and worksites. They are health educators, health promoters, nutritionists, physical fitness experts, and lifestyle change coaches. These experts can help those persons at risk of developing a chronic disease, such as type 2 diabetes, to reduce their risk as well as reverse the condition through a structured comprehensive lifestyle change program.

The Plan is the vision of the Mississippi health officer, a medical doctor, and the Mississippi State Board of Health. The Board's membership, which is appointed by the governor, does not adequately reflect the State's population or its pressing public health needs. For instance, although Mississippi is 37 percent Black and 51 percent female, the Board is comprised of 99 percent Whites, of whom about 73 percent are men.

Furthermore, the membership is composed almost exclusively of clinical professionals, especially physicians, who account for 54 percent. Other members include a nurse, physical therapist, communications professor, a former state representative, a banker, and the president of a pecan company. A previous board member was a general manager of an electric power company.[154] The Board excludes primary prevention professionals, who are experts in obesity and chronic disease prevention.

In addition, the state legislature and governor have responded to Mississippi's continuous public health crisis with an elaborate plan to expand the State's medical care industry. In 2012, Governor Phil Bryant signed into law the *Mississippi Health Care Industry Zone Act* to promote the growth of the industry, one of the fastest growing industries in the State.

Like the *Mississippi Health Plan,* the Act will create more clinical based jobs but not prevention centered ones. It will certainly increase the profit margins of medical care facilities through generous incentives such as tax deductions and exemptions. It will ensure that Mississippians have greater access to more diagnostic tests, biotechnology, new and expensive drug medications, acute care, and hospital beds to treat preventable chronic conditions, but unfortunately it will do absolutely nothing to address obesity, prevent chronic diseases, and achieve wellness.

The Way Forward

If the state of Mississippi is serious about reducing rates of obesity, chronic diseases, and deaths, it will need to make disease prevention the main focus of its health plan. This approach will necessitate various state programs working with businesses, community organizations, local governments and the federal government to create residential and work environments that promote and sustain healthy living. It also will require a large and diverse public health workforce capable of developing and managing public health programs designed to address disease prevention and wellness, which are objectives of the Affordable Care Act (ACA) prevention provisions.

The ACA is the first federal initiative to make chronic disease prevention the central focus of health care in the U.S. Federal agencies are providing funding, technical support, and guidance to state and local governments and employers to reduce the burden of chronic diseases. Its goal is to implement proven community-based programs that are designed to prevent diseases such as obesity, cancer, type 2 diabetes, heart disease and stroke.[(155)] A variety of prevention-centered programs are being rolled out, such as the healthy lifestyle change intervention program for Medicaid beneficiaries, the National Diabetes Prevention Program, and a program to utilize community health workers to promote healthy behaviors and outcomes among poor populations. Also, it provides support for worksite wellness programs within small and large businesses.

Additionally, about $270 million has been appropriated for the recruitment and training of the U.S. public health work force.[(156)] The aim is to increase the number of public health professionals through a number of training, recruitment, and retention programs.

Currently, Mississippi has received about $179.6 million, from the ACA's Prevention and Public Health Fund. Twelve federally funded health centers that provide medical services for over 300,000 Mississippi residents have received $55.2 million to expand 'services' and establish new health center locations.[157]

If the State continues to take an absolutely clinical approach to health care, Mississippians, especially Blacks, will persist in experiencing the worse health in the nation. Rather than resist the ACA, the State's leaders should expand Medicaid and implement many of the ACA prevention based programs. Furthermore, Mississippians must begin electing public servants who genuinely care about their well-being and quality of life and who will place the public's health above party politics. Furthermore, health insurance executives who are serious about reducing medical claims associated with preventable diseases should work with in-network medical providers (obstetrician and gynecologists, family nurse practitioners, and pediatricians) to promote (1) the health benefits of breast-feeding and (2) breast-feeding benefit coverage among their patient/member populations. In addition, they could substantially reduce the prevalence of hypertension, high cholesterol, heart disease, and type 2 diabetes if they would make the National Diabetes Prevention Program and the Ornish Spectrum Programs for Prevention, and Reversing Heart Disease covered preventive health benefits. Adopting these measures would be a major game changer in the health care system, and it would significantly improve the overall well-being of Mississippi and the nation.

PART III

Congenial Soil

"The seeds of a plant are carried in all directions; but they can only live and grow if they fall on congenial soil."

The Seed and Soil Hypothesis by Stephen Paget

Chapter 6

Preventing Type 1 Diabetes

Type 1 diabetes mellitus is an autoimmune disease caused by the destruction of the insulin producing beta cells located in the islets of the pancreas. The pancreatic islet cells are composed of the alpha and beta cells that produce insulin. The antibodies that attack the islet cells are referred to as auto-antibodies because they attack the body's own cells.

The islet cell auto-antibodies are often predictive of those individuals who will eventually develop the disease. Islet cell auto-antibodies often precede the development of type 1 diabetes and are present in most individuals who have type 1 diabetes. These islet autoantibodies are known as islet autoimmunity.

Type 1 diabetes usually develops in children, adolescents, and young adults. In most children it manifests around 2 and 3 years of age.[(158)] The significant increase of the disease over a relatively short period of time suggests that controllable environmental factors (triggers) may be contributing to the increase among children who are genetically predisposed. Some environmental factors linked to type 1 diabetes are: viruses, mode of delivery, bodyweight, and infant nutrition.

Breastfeeding – A Preventive Factor

Nearly 30 years ago, Scandinavian researchers reported that children who were born when breastfeeding was the societal norm were less likely to develop type 1 diabetes compared with children who were born when formula feeding was more common. This suggests that breastfeeding acts as a preventive factor and formula feeding a risk factor.[159] Since then additional studies from around the globe have validated that breastfeeding offers protection against type 1 diabetes disease.[160]

The duration of breastfeeding and whether or not an infant is exclusively breast-fed may affect the child's risk for type 1 diabetes. Studies have shown that the longer a child is breast-fed the less likely it is to develop the disease.[167-168]

The protection may be derived from breast milk's antibacterial and antiviral antibodies that enable the infant's body to withstand numerous infections such as E. coli, Salmonella, Shigella, Streptococcus, polio virus, Rubella virus, herpes simplex virus, mumps, and pneumonia.[169]

Breast milk significantly reduces the occurrence, duration, and/or severity of the following health conditions among infants and young children: obesity, Haemophilus influenza,[170-171] pneumonia,[172] middle ear infections,[173-174] cholera, Respiratory syncytial virus,[175-180] urinary tract infections,[181] gastrointestinal infections,[182-184] bacterial meningitis,[185] Streptococcus pneumoniae,[186] Sudden Infant Death Syndrome (SIDS),[187-188] Crohn's disease,[189-190] celia disease,[191-192] leukemia, lymphoma,[193-194] ulcerative colitis,[195] and diarrhea.[196-197]

It also is composed of protective factors, such as bifidus growth factor that protects a child's immune system from various viruses. Bifidus growth stimulating factor protects against enterepathogens, a microorganism that causes disease in the intestine.[198]

Breast milk also contains the epidermal growth factor, which is more prominent in colostrum (early breast milk). Epidermal growth factor is responsible for absorbing nutrients, secreting waste,[199] and stimulating the production of the gastrointestinal lining and intestinal epithelium, as well as strengthening the human gastrointestinal mucosal barrier to antigens.[200-201]

The gastrointestinal tract is the largest mucosal surface (the thin layer that lines body cavities and passages) within the human body. It is in constant contact with various micro-organisms and dietary antigens (substances that cause the immune system to manufacture antibodies against it) that may play an integral role in the development of type 1 diabetes.[202-203] The gastrointestinal tract is especially vulnerable in infants because it is in the developing stage.

Fortunately, nature has designed the mother's mature milk and colostrum with other powerful weapons known as secretory immunoglobulins (antibodies) that protect the newborn's immature gastrointestinal and immune systems from microbial infections. They include secretory IgM (SIgM), secretory IgD (SIgD), secretory IgG (SIgG) and secretory IgA (SIgA).[204] Of these 4 types, SIgA is the predominant antibody in human milk.

SIgA is secreted throughout the first year of lactation.[205] An exclusively breast-fed baby receives between 0.5g and 1g of SIgA antibodies each day.[206] SIgA is the first line of defense against pathogens as it protects the newborn's mucosal membranes, respiratory system, urogenital system, and gastrointestinal system.[207] It prevents enteropathogens from attaching to the cellular covering of the gut in breastfeeding infants,[208] and it protects against dietary antigens.

This is important because enterovirus infections, which are the most frequent viruses responsible for human diseases,[209] are associated with the development of type 1 diabetes.[210-212] Enterovirus infections occur more frequently in children who have type 1 diabetes.[213] It is suggested that enterovirus infections may trigger an autoimmune reaction that causes the destruction of the beta cells. The infections have been found in the mucous membrane of the small intestine of type 1 diabetic patients.[214]

As stated earlier, the newborn's gastrointestinal tract is not fully developed (*complete intestinal closure*), and it does not completely develop until 6 to 9 months of age.[215-216] Prior to maturation the infant's gut is porous, which makes it vulnerable to foreign dietary antigens (substances that cause the immune system to produce antibodies against it) that can pass through and cause an autoimmune response in genetically predisposed children. Therefore, postponing the introduction of foreign dietary antigens until the infant is 9 months or older may allow its own digestive system to become fully operative and defend it against dietary antigens.

According to authors Riordan and Auerbach, feeding an infant "exclusive breast milk facilitates the maturation of the intestinal barrier and provides exogenous passive barrier…"[217] Although breast milk offers protection, dairy based formula has been reported to increase the risk of gastrointestinal infections in newborns.

Cow's Milk

Cow's milk is the first and most frequent dietary antigen that an infant's gastrointestinal system encounters.[218-219] The majority of international studies have found that when infants prematurely consume dairy, specifically cow's milk, their risk increases for developing type 1 diabetes.

Finland researchers were the first to establish that early introduction of dairy products is independently associated with type 1 diabetes.[220] They reported that the occurrence of the disease was doubled in children who consumed dairy foods at less than 2 months of age. However, the risk of developing the disease was lower among children who had been breast-fed more than 4 months compared with those who were breast-fed less than 2 months or not at all.

In another study, Brazilian researchers found a relationship between the timing of dairy consumption and type 1 diabetes. Children who consumed cow's milk during the first 7 days of life were at an increased risk of developing type 1 diabetes compared with children who had been exclusively breast-fed longer and who consumed cow's milk later in life.[221] Additional studies have reported that delaying dairy milk until **after** the first 3 months of life may reduce the risk of developing type 1 diabetes.[222-225]

It is suggested that one or more of the five principal proteins (beta-lactoglobulin, beta-casein, a-lactalbumin, bovine serum albumin, and globulin) found in cow's milk acts as a dietary antigen that triggers an autoimmune response in vulnerable children that leads to the destruction of the pancreatic beta-cells, which are responsible for producing insulin.

Substantially higher levels of antibodies to cow's milk proteins have been found in children who were diagnosed with type 1 diabetes.[226-237]

In response to the mounting evidence linking cow's milk to type 1 diabetes, in 1994, the American Academy of Pediatrics Work Group on Cow's Milk Protein and Diabetes Mellitus reported: [238]

> It has been known for several years that children with insulin dependent diabetes mellitus have an increased frequency of antibodies to a variety of cow's milk proteins, which is particularly evident in those with early onset type 1 diabetes. The avoidance of cow's milk protein for the first several months of life may reduce the later development of type 1 diabetes or delay its onset in susceptible individuals.

The Work Group recommended that breast milk be the primary nutritional source for the first year of life and that families who are genetically predisposed to type 1 diabetes, e.g. a sibling, avoid dairy milk and its food products during the first year. It further stated that soy milk based formula was linked to type 1 diabetes and should be avoided. However, it identified no evidence to substantiate this claim and recommendation. The author has found no studies that reported such a relationship. In addition to dairy foods, the timing of solid foods has been linked to an increased risk of obesity, type 2 diabetes, and type 1 diabetes among young children.

The Timing of Solid Foods

Rapid weight gain during the first 3 months of life is linked to obesity in childhood and adulthood.[239-241] Overweight children have a significant risk of developing a number of chronic diseases such as asthma, hyperlipidemia, hypertension, and diabetes.[242-243]

In an effort to prevent childhood obesity, the Expert Consultation of the World Health Organization recommends that solid foods be introduced at 6 months in conjunction with continued breastfeeding.[244] The American Academy of Pediatrics Committee on Nutrition, and the American Academy of Pediatrics Section on Breastfeeding recommend delaying solid foods until a minimum of 4 months but preferably until 6 months of age.[245-246] Research findings support recommendations to delay solid foods until a child is between 4 months and 6 months of age and preferably introduce the foods while the child is still being breast-fed.

Boston's Children Hospital researchers investigated the diet of newborns over a period of 3 years to determine if a link exists between the timing of solid food introduction and obesity.[247] They concluded that infants who consumed solid foods **before** 4 months of age experienced a 6-fold increased risk of being obese at 3 years of age.

Among formula-fed children, the risk was reduced by nearly half when foods were introduced at 6 months of age. In contrast, the timing of solid foods did not increase the risk among children who were breast-fed for 4 months or longer. In a Cornell Universty study, researchers found the timing of solid foods did not cause an increased weight gain among infants who were breast-fed beyond 5 months.[248]

Since 1994, University of Colorado's Diabetes Autoimmunity Study in the Young (DAISY) has examined possible environmental triggers of type 1 diabetes among children who are genetically susceptible to the disease. Among other findings, they have reported that children who were genetically predisposed to type 1 diabetes and who consumed solid foods and cow's milk before 3 months of age had an increased risk of developing the disease.[249]

Another DAISY study showed that children, genetically susceptible to type 1 diabetes, who initially consumed rice cereals prior to 3 months of age or at 7 months or older experienced an increased risk of developing islet autoimmunity (precursor to type 1 diabetes) compared with those who consumed cereals between 4 and 6 months of age. However, children who were still being breast-fed when they were exposed to cereals experienced a reduced risk. The decreased risk among breast-fed children was independent of the child's age when it initially consumed the cereals.[250]

Early consumption of gluten foods may be a risk factor for children genetically predisposed to developing type 1 diabetes. Findings from a German study showed that children who consumed gluten foods before 3 months of age experienced a significantly greater risk of developing islet autoimmunity compared with children who were introduced to the foods between 3.1 and 6 months of age. The researchers found no increased risk among children who consumed gluten foods after 6 months of age. Also, children who were genetically predisposed to developing type 1 diabetes had significantly lower periods of breast-feeding compared with those who were not genetically susceptible.[251] The premature consumption of gluten foods may increase the risk of developing gastrointestinal infections, which are associated with type 1 diabetes.

Gastrointestinal Infections

A DAISY study reported that gastrointestinal infections were significantly associated with an increase in islet autoimmunity among children who initially consumed gluten foods (wheat or barley) before the age of 4 months or after 6 months of age. Each gastrointestinal infection was related to a 37 percent increased probability of islet autoimmunity developing among children who consumed wheat less than 4 months of age, and a 12 percent increased probability among children who consumed gluten foods at 7 months or older. On the other hand, children who consumed gluten foods between 4 months and 6 months of age did not experience any increased risk. The researchers stated:[252]

> Wheat protein antigens can induce an inflammatory response in the gut and so could prime the immune system for a detrimental response to infection with a viral agent.

Delaying the gradual introduction of gluten foods until 4 to 6 months of age and while breastfeeding may also prevent celiac disease. [253-254]

The First Building Blocks

A mother's gastrointestinal tract (maternal gut) is designed to protect her newborn's immune system as it is being born. The gut is host to the largest and most complex assortment of micro-organisms, known as gut microbiota.[255] Gut bacteria promote intestinal homeostasis (internal stability), stimulates development of the immune system, and acts as a barrier against pathogens. [256] Katrina Ray of Nature Reviews Gastroenterology & Hepatology wrote:[257]

> ...our mothers play a vital part in providing the first 'building blocks' for the development of our resident microbiota, jump-starting the stepwise colonization of our intestines and the rest of the human body through skin-to-skin contact and breastfeeding. Once the gut microbiota becomes established and stabilized by age 2–3 years, these bacteria have a crucial role in nutrition and health.

Mode of Delivery

One of the foremost determining factors of the gut microbiota is the mode of delivery. There is an important difference between the compositions of gut microbiota in infants delivered vaginally and those born through a Cesarean section (C-section). In other words, the manner in which a baby enters the world affects the development of its immune system. [258-260]

As a newborn passes through the birth canal it comes in direct contact with its mother's gut microbiota.[261] Intestinal microbiota makeup of the vaginally born infant is quantitatively and qualitatively similar to that of its mother's vaginal microbiota.[262-263] The C-section born infant has a different microbial composition.[264]

The infant born through C-section is exposed to microbes, such as Staphylococcus, that are similar to those found on the skin.[265] It also is exposed to bacteria that exist within birthing facilities and on medical staff.[(266)] The C-section delivery disturbs normal colonization of the infant gut by preventing exposure to the mother's microbes. This disruption may be a contributing factor in the increased rate of type 1 diabetes among infants born through C-sections.

As an example, women who reside in Newfoundland and Labrador, Canada have one of the world's highest rates of repeat C-sections, and their children have one of the highest rates of type 1 diabetes in the world. Canadian researchers found that the disease was significantly higher among children 0–15 years of age and who were born through the C-section mode of delivery.[(267)]

An analysis of 20 studies from 15 predominantly European countries involving over 9000 children showed a 20 percent increase in the risk of developing type 1 diabetes among children who were born through C-section.[(268)] Infant birth weight, maternal age, genetic predisposition, or breastfeeding status did not influence the relationship between C-section delivery and type 1 diabetes.

Findings of German researchers showed the risk of developing type 1 diabetes by age 12 was significantly higher in children who were delivered by C-sections. Within 10 years, the rate of progression from the development of islet auto-antibodies to clinical type 1 diabetes among children who were born through C-sections was 57 percent compared with 28 percent of those children born vaginally.[(269)]

C-section delivery also has been linked to a 20 percent increase in childhood asthma,[(270)] hospitalization for asthma, food allergy/food atopy,[(271-272)] as well as an increase in allergic rhinoconjunctivitis.[(273)]

C-section delivery is the 2nd most common surgical procedure in the U.S. with 1.3 million procedures occurring annually. The current rate is 32.8 percent, a huge increase from 22.8 percent in 1989[(274)] and 4.5 percent in 1965.[(275)] Black women account for the highest rate of C-section deliveries followed by White women and Hispanic women. New Jersey has the highest rates followed by Florida, Mississippi, and Louisiana.[276]

Interestingly, in addition to having one of the highest C-section rates, Mississippi has the lowest breastfeeding rates in the nation. Rochelle Fields, a lactation counselor in Mississippi, believes the problem is driven by lack of education, promotion, and medical profits:

> Women are not being exposed to breastfeeding information or images in clinics, hospitals, government health offices or physicians' offices where they receive maternal and child health care and resources. Consequently, I meet many clients who have never heard of breastfeeding or ever seen anyone breastfeeding. They deliver at hospitals where nurses often give them wrong information, e.g. breast milk and formula are the same. I have to dispel the misinformation or it will pass on to other women who will accept it as the truth and choose not to breastfeed. Many employers do not support employees who breastfeed, which discourages initiation and shortens duration. Many of my clients are having unnecessary C-sections because they don't realize the dangers associated with this procedure. They are often encouraged by their physicians to have the procedure because it fits nicely into their busy schedules. And it's a cash cow for physicians and birthing facilities.

Other Nutritional Factors

Aside from exclusive breastfeeding, and the postponement of solid foods, some dietary supplements may help reduce the risk of children developing type 1 diabetes. Cod liver oil may offer protection against the disease. Cod liver oil contains omega 3 fatty acids, and vitamins A and D. It has been reported to significantly promote bone health and reduce upper respiratory infections among young children.[277] Findings from various studies have shown that genetically susceptible children who consumed cod liver oil within the first year, specifically 7 – 12 months of life, experienced a significantly reduced risk of developing type 1 diabetes.[278-279]

Pregnant women who take cod liver oil may provide passive protection against type 1 diabetes to their newborns.[280] Also, women who consumed vitamin D during pregnancy have been shown to significantly reduce the risk of their newborn developing islet cell auto-antibodies.[281]

Vitamin D consumed during childhood has been shown to reduce the risk of type 1 diabetes.[282] Vitamin D deficiency may be a risk factor as young adults, children, and adolescents who have type 1 diabetes have been found to be deficient in vitamin D compared with those who do not have the disease.[283-284]

Bodyweight

As indicated earlier, the early introduction of solid foods can lead to excessive weight gain, and infant weight gain is associated with the development of diabetes. Breastfeeding can help control the amount of weight a baby gains. Breast-fed babies have an innate ability to meet their nutritional needs by self-regulating their caloric intake.[285] Breast-fed babies grow at a slower rate than formula-fed babies, who are more likely to become obese[286-288] and develop type 2 diabetes.[289-290]

As one study showed, during the first 3 months of life, breast-fed and formula-fed newborns had the same body weight, but during the next 9 months the breast-fed babies were leaner, and they did not gain weight as fast as formula-fed infants.[291] At 4 months of age, breast-fed babies consume a lower volume of breast milk and fewer calories compared with formula-fed babies.[292]

In summary, breastfeeding is the best protection against many childhood diseases, including type 1 diabetes and rare illnesses, e.g. acute lymphoblastic, myeloid leukemia,[(293-297)] Hodgkin's disease,[(298-299)] and neuroblastoma.[(300)] Parents should seriously consider delaying the introduction of solid foods, especially those containing gluten, until 4 to 6 months and preferably while the baby is still being breast-fed.

CHAPTER 7

Preventing & Reversing Type 2 Diabetes

"Do you want to live or do you want to die?"

There is a striking physical contrast in Lisa Whittington from 8 years ago and today. She is an energetic and youthful looking middle age woman who has no resemblance to the woman who once lived without any consideration for her health.

Her former unhealthy lifestyle caught up with her in 2006 when she was diagnosed with type 2 diabetes. At the time of the diagnosis, she was 5'4", and weighed 263 pounds. Her glucose level was over 300 and her blood pressure was 160/100.

Lisa also has a family history of heart disease and diabetes. Her father died of heart disease at 58 years of age. At age 51, one of her brothers died of diabetes. Her deceased mother had late onset type 2 diabetes. Family history was not enough to motivate Lisa to take the necessary steps to prevent diabetes from occurring. No, it would take extreme foot pain to put her on the path to wellness:

> I developed severe neuropathy in my feet; it was so painful I could barely walk or touch my feet. So, I visited the doctor who informed me that I had type 2 diabetes. I re-

> member him asking, 'do you want to live or do you want to die?' 'I'm going to get busy living,' I said. 'Then you got to lose weight,' he told me.

For 2 -3 months Lisa took no course of action, but later she began to become gradually active:

> I began swimming laps about 4 times a week. My former husband played golf so I walked the golf course while he drove the buggy. I went to the tread mill about every day. My weight dropped to about 230 within 7 months, but I had not made any dietary changes at that point."

Even though she lost weight, the pain in her feet did not improve. It was so painful eventually she stopped exercising.

In 2007, Lisa began volunteering at a 12 step program. One day the manager received a call from his son who had recently opened a vitamin and nutritional supplement store for which he needed assistance. She was asked to help out. While working there, the owner took a picture of Lisa for the company's website. When she saw herself she was horrified.

> "I thought, what is a girl like me doing in a place like this? I was out of shape, fat, diabetic and hypertensive. I was the poster child of unhealthy living. That's when I made the commitment to finally get busy making a healthy life style change.

Lisa began walking around her neighborhood every afternoon. She joined the YMCA where she took aerobic classes. A month later, she began walking 2 miles every day. By 2009, she was weighing 217 lbs. During the next year, her weight began to fluctuate, but her glucose level remained high. Although Lisa had become physically active, she had refused to make any dietary changes.

> I was eating McDonalds' double quarter pounder 3-4 times a week and drinking 4-5 Diet Cokes a day. When I wasn't eating McDonald's, I ate Pizza Hut's pizza or fried chicken. I also drank a lot of sweet tea but absolutely no water.

Her understanding of food and disease drastically changed upon reading a book about processed foods and chronic diseases. It was at this point that she made a commitment to changing her diet:

> On December 7, 1998, I became sober, and I never looked back, but I would have killed you for a Diet Coke. I believe I was addicted to the aspartame. On August 11, 2010, I drank my last Diet Coke. I said no more. Reluctantly, I began drinking water. I counted every single day that I did not have a Diet Coke. The days turned into weeks and the weeks into months. I decided that if I can stop drinking Diet Coke, I could also stop eating fast foods. None of this happened over night; I targeted one addiction at a time. In September of 2011, I had my last double quarter pounder.

She began consuming local or raw honey, Bragg's apple cider vinegar, and lemon juice. She replaced artificial sweeteners with Stevia (a plant based natural sugar).

> I no longer eat fast foods and processed foods. I eat grass fed red meat occasionally and poultry that was raised

> cage free and without hormones and antibiotics. I am still learning to read nutritional labels.

After getting control of her diet, she intensified her physical activity level. She increased her walking to 3 miles a day and joined a long term boot camp. Over the past several years, she has competed in several 5-K walks. In one competition, she placed 2nd and her finishing time was 39 minutes. She has placed 1st in two previous competitions and has had numerous 2nd places. "My goal has always been to simply cross the finish line," she said.

Currently, Lisa weighs 178 lbs and has a goal of reaching 150 lbs. She feels healthy for the first time in many years, and she owes it all to her lifestyle change:

> When I started on this path, my glucose level was between 340 and 289, but today it's between 120 and 130, and my blood pressure is 128/78. I never took drug medications because I did not have medical insurance and could not afford to pay. Knowing what I now know about prescription drugs, I am glad that I did not take them, and I would choose natural alternatives again if I had to do it over. The neuropathy isn't as intense but it has not gone away. If I had known I was going to live this long, I would have taken better care of myself but even at 52, I feel like I am coming into my own and there is more wellness and living to come.

Type 2 Diabetes Mellitus

An unhealthy lifestyle and obesity are common among most individuals who have type 2 diabetes or who are pre-diabetic. Once a disease of the elderly, rich, and Western nations, type 2 diabetes is expanding rapidly among young and poor populations and nations in the East. Asia, for example, now accounts for 60 percent of diabetics in the world.[301] Diabetes affects approximately 285 million people worldwide, and it is expected to reach 438 million by 2030.

Within the U.S., an estimated 26 million people have type 2 diabetes mellitus, according to the most recent data. Moreover, 79 million Americans have prediabetes.[302] When compared with Whites, the risk of being diagnosed with diabetes is 18 percent, 66 percent, and 77 percent higher among Asians, Hispanics, and Blacks, respectively.[303]

Type 2 diabetes is a major cause of heart disease, stroke, and kidney failure. It is the leading cause of lower extremity amputations, which are more prevalent in southern states. For instance, Medicaid beneficiaries in Mississippi, Arkansas, Louisiana, and Texas, and southern Oklahoma have the highest rates of diabetes-related amputations.[304]

Lifestyle Change

A growing body of evidence has established that the vast majority of diabetes cases can be prevented[305-311] and reversed[312-316] through lifestyle change programs designed to help individuals to change unhealthy diets and behaviors that place them at risk for developing the disease.

Noted physician and researcher Neal Barnard is leading a national movement to make lifestyle change programs the new model for treating type 2 diabetes. His approach is based upon a number of racially diverse studies that established the effectiveness of treating the disease with a plant-based diet (vegan) and exercise. In fact, his vegan diet has been reported to be more effective than the American Diabetes Association (ADA) recommended diet, which contains meat and dairy, in treating the disease.[317-319]

Several studies compared the two diets and found nearly twice as many individuals who consumed the low-fat, high fiber vegan diet experienced substantial reductions in glycemic index, body weight, LDL cholesterol and total cholesterol levels, average HbA1c points, diabetes medication dosage and urinary albumin.

In general, adopting a healthy diet, exercise, and tobacco cessation is a more effective strategy to prevent the disease than taking diabetes medication, which has been demonstrated by several studies, including the National Diabetes Prevention Program.

The study on which the National Diabetes Prevention Program is based showed that individuals who had pre-diabetes but who followed a low-calorie, low-fat, high fiber diet and performed moderate intensity exercises, such as brisk walking, were more successful at preventing the onset of type 2 diabetes and metabolic syndrome than those individuals who consumed Metformin, the popular diabetes drug. [320-321]

The lifestyle change group reduced its incidence of type 2 diabetes by 58 percent compared with the Metformin group's 31 percent. Although Metformin and the lifestyle change therapy were equally effective in returning the participants' normal fasting glucose values, the lifestyle change program proved to be more effective at re-establishing normal post-load glucose values and for a longer period of time. After 3 years, the prevalence of the metabolic syndrome **increased** from 54 percent to 55 percent among the Metformin group, but it **decreased** from 51 percent to 43 percent among the lifestyle change group. Overall, the lifestyle change program proved to be more effective and feasible.

The lifestyle change program was more effective than Metformin because it targeted the underlying causes (risk factors) associated with type 2 diabetes. Until underlying risk factors are changed or eliminated, type 2 diabetes or some other chronic condition will usually develop and/or worsen.

Diabetes Risk Factors

Race and Age

National diabetes organizations have a tendency to include age (45+) and race (Blacks, Asians, Pacific Islanders, and Native Americans) as risk factors for type 2 diabetes. This is misleading because research has shown that an unhealthy lifestyle is usually responsible for the high prevalence of type 2 diabetes among all groups of people. In fact, when other racial groups make healthy lifestyle changes they experience similar health outcomes as Whites. Older individuals also benefit by adopting healthy lifestyle changes.

There are six proven factors that an ambulatory (able to walk) individual of any race and age can change to prevent developing pre-diabetes and type 2 diabetes: overweight/obesity, diet, physical inactivity, tobacco use, and gestational diabetes.

Abdominal obesity

Obesity is the strongest modifiable risk factor for type 2 diabetes. So, maintaining a healthy body weight throughout adulthood is vital to preventing the disease.[322] The worse place to develop excess weight is the abdominal section because it greatly increases the risk of developing the disease.[323-326]

This is because the fat in the tissues causes an imbalance of insulin known as insulin resistance. Fortunately, the fat can be eliminated through abdominal exercises and a diet low in fat and simple carbohydrates, especially sugar and HFCS. Weight loss in the abdominal section can return glucose to a healthy level and help prevent the disease.

High rates of abdominal obesity helps to explain the high prevalence of diabetes among Asian populations, who tend to have lower overall obesity rates but greater abdominal fat. At every BMI level or waist circumference, Asians have a greater amount of abdominal fat than Whites, according to several multi-racial studies.[327-329]

According to Dr. Frank Hu, a professor of nutrition and epidemiology at Harvard University, the risk of type 2 diabetes begins at a lower body weight and younger age among Asians compared with Whites. ".., even a modest amount of weight gain during adulthood substantially increases the risk of diabetes in Asians, wrote Dr. Hu. He points out that Asians are more likely to have abdominal obesity and less muscle mass that leads to an increased predisposition for insulin resistance.[330]

It is worth noting that type 2 diabetes is more prevalent among urban

Asians and Asian Americans compared with those who reside in rural Asian communities and maintain a traditional lifestyle. This further suggests that lifestyle is the major determinant of type 2 diabetes.

Additionally, people who are genetically predisposed to the condition and regularly consume a typical Western diet, specifically processed meats, red meats, and heme iron, may have an even greater risk of becoming diabetic, according to Harvard University researchers[(331)]:

> ..., preserving, cooking, and processing these foods generate certain types of preservatives, additives, or other chemicals such as advanced glycation and lipoxidation end products that have toxic effect on beta cells or induce insulin resistance.

Diet

Consuming a low carbohydrate, high fiber, and primarily fresh (whole) foods diet is essential to eliminating risk factors that often lead to metabolic syndrome and type 2 diabetes. For instance, replacing whole dairy food with low fat dairy is a simple but effective dietary change that can help prevent diabetes. Several studies have reported that consuming low-fat dairy, e.g. yogurt, reduces the risk of developing type 2 diabetes.[(332-334)]

A diet high in red meat, especially processed meats, considerably increases the risk.[(335-341)] Meat is high in heme-iron. A high consumption of heme-iron is associated with an increased risk of developing the disease.[(342-344)] For instance, pregnant women who consumed high levels of meat before and during the early stages of pregnancy had a substantially increased risk of developing gestational diabetes.[(345-347)]

Plants are a healthier source of iron, known as non-heme iron. Some foods high in iron include: nuts, spinach, broccoli, Blackstrap molasses, tofu, legumes, raisins, and dates). Vitamin C foods (oranges, grapefruits, tomatoes, broccoli and strawberries) help increase absorption of plant based iron foods.[(348)]

Eating a primarily plant based diet improves levels of HDL, triglycerides, glucose, blood pressure, waist circumference, and reduces the risk of developing metabolic syndrome.[349] For instance, consuming a lot of blueberries, strawberries, and especially pears and apples, may significantly lower the risk of developing type 2 diabetes.[350]

Apples also are linked to a reduction of other diseases such as asthma, thrombotic stroke, ischemic heart disease, and prostate and lung cancers. Eating large amounts of apples and onions may reduce the risk of dying from ischemic heart disease.[351]

As reported earlier, consuming a lot of foods and beverages that are high in sugar and high fructose corn syrup are a leading cause of abdominal obesity, hypertension, metabolic syndrome, and type 2 diabetes. Substantially reducing the intake of sweetened beverages is critical to preventing type 2 diabetes.

Drinking sweetened beverages quickly raises blood glucose and insulin levels and contributes to a high dietary glycemic load[352] causing glucose intolerance and insulin resistance, especially within overweight and obese individuals.

Adults who have type 2 diabetes tend to consume high levels of sweetened beverages.[353] A large number of studies have found a positive relationship between type 2 diabetes and sweetened beverages. Among the findings, people who consumed 2 or more soft drinks or juice beverages per week had a 42 percent and 29 percent, respectively, increased risk of developing diabetes,[354] weight gain, and metabolic syndrome. [355]

A deficiency in magnesium may increase the risk of developing type 2 diabetes[356-358] and of type 2 diabetics dying of heart failure.[359] Magnesium, a mineral found in many foods, is important to blood glucose control. Some magnesium rich foods include: whole grains, beans, green leafy vegetables and nuts, such as peanut butter.[360-361] Eating nuts or peanut butter 5 times per week may lower the risk of developing type 2 diabetes.[362]

Individuals who have a high risk of developing type 2 diabetes and are severely vitamin D deficient may have an increased risk of coronary artery disease,[363] and cardiovascular death.[364] Having a healthy vitamin D level reduces the risk of developing hypertension,[365-366] prediabetes,[367] and type 2 diabetes.[368]

Physical Activity

Regular physical activity substantially reduces the risk of developing the disease.[369-372] Exercise programs that include aerobic exercise and/or resistance training may greatly reduce HbA(1c) among type 2 diabetic patients.[373-375]

Moderate intense resistant training improves insulin sensitivity, glycemia, and lipids in type 2 diabetic patients.[376] Aerobic exercise alone or combined with resistance training can improve glycemic control, systolic blood pressure, triglycerides, and waist circumference among type 2 diabetic patients.[377] Physical activity does not need to be strenuous. Simple brisk walking may reduce the risk of developing the disease.[378] Yoga also has been reported to improve glycemic control,[379] body weight, blood pressure, insulin, and triglycerides of individuals at high risk for type 2 diabetes.[380]

Cigarettes

Smoking or being exposed to secondhand smoke should be avoided as each increases the risk of developing type 2 diabetes.[381] Smoking also has a negative effect on insulin sensitivity and exacerbates metabolic control.[382]

Gestational Diabetes

There are some steps a pregnant woman can take to reduce the risk of developing gestational diabetes. Between 5 percent and 10 percent of women who have gestational diabetes tend to progress to type 2 diabetes immediately following their pregnancies.[383] In the U.S., gestational diabetes is more common among Black women, who have the highest rates of progression to type 2 diabetes.[384]

Obesity is the most important risk factor a woman can change to prevent type 2 diabetes, and it is the leading cause of the type 2 diabetes among Black women.[385] Therefore it is vital that pregnant women maintain a healthy body weight during pregnancy and preferably during preconception.

Being physically active reduces the risk of developing gestational diabetes during pregnancy. In one study, a group of pregnant women who performed high levels of physical activity before and after pregnancy were successful at lowering their risk of developing gestational diabetes.[386]

In contrast, another group of women who were inactive during the early stages of their pregnancies increased their risk of developing gestational diabetes.[387] Being active as early as a year before pregnancy may substantially reduce the risk of developing diabetes.[388]

Women who develop gestational diabetes may prevent its progression to type 2 diabetes through breastfeeding, which has been shown to reduce the prevalence of persistent hyperglycemia[389-390] and postpartum maternal glucose tolerance. In one study, women who breast-fed delayed type 2 diabetes by an average of 12.2 years compared with 2.3 years for those who formula-fed. Those women who breast-fed more than 3 months had the lowest risk of developing the disease.[391]

Three months of breastfeeding has been shown to improve glucose metabolism and increase in HDL cholesterol levels among mothers with gestational diabetes.[392] Women who exclusively breast-fed improved their fasting glucose and lowered insulin levels between 6 and 9 weeks after giving birth compared with those who primarily formula-fed.[393]

Type 2 diabetes is primarily rising because healthy lifestyles have been replaced by unhealthy ones that lead to obesity, especially abdominal obesity. The most effective approach to reducing pre-diabetes and type 2 diabetes is through lifestyle change programs that target diet, physical activity, tobacco, breastfeeding, among others.

CHAPTER 8

Preventing & Reversing Heart Disease

There are no guarantees, but we should at a minimum try to stay healthy for as long as we can.

Don Williams

From his slender appearance, you would never expect Don Williams, a Black middle age male, to have ever experienced a health condition. Not long ago, Don's blood pressure began to increase, which adversely affected his health and quality of life.

He had gained about 10-15 lbs. The extra weight caused him to snore at night, and his shirt collar size jumped from a 15 ½" to 17". He realized that he did not look or feel as well as he used to. His energy level was significantly lower, and his blood pressure higher, 140/85. Rather than take hypertensive medication and buy new dress shirts, he decided he needed to make a lifestyle change:

In 2011, I began changing my diet. I cut high fructose corn syrup out of my diet. It's in most if not all processed foods and drinks so I switched to 100% whole fruit juice, which costs more money but is healthy and taste better. One of the hardest things I had to do was giving up sweet tea, which is a preferred beverage by many Mississippians. I was drinking 3-4 glasses at dinner, but now I drink water. That was one of the key things in helping me to lose weight. I also cut out the dairy foods, including milk, processed foods, junk foods, frozen, canned, etc. I switched to eating more whole fresh foods. I began juicing vegetables 3-4 years ago. One of the big differences with juicing and eating fresh produce was the regularity. Before the dietary change, my bowels moved once or twice a week to every day. I began taking 2000 IU of Vitamin D3 supplement, 1000 mg of vitamin C 1000, Bragg's apple cider vinegar a couple times a week. I had always exercised, but I began doing it every day. My exercise routine usually involves stretching, pushups and other cardio, jump rump, and I ride my bike. I also targeted my midsection with pushups to tone up my abdominal section.

Since implementing his lifestyle change, Don has lost 3 inches from his waistline, and his overall bodyweight is now 165 lbs. He also has reduced the excess weight in his abdominal section. His neck size has dropped; so, he can wear his old dress shirts again. His blood pressure is consistently 120/70.

Don believes that we all can take steps toward improving our cardiovascular health. His advice is to stop smoking, reduce alcohol consumption or stop drinking. Reduce the amount of dairy and fried foods. Drastically decrease sweetened beverage consumption while increasing the intake of fresh fruits, vegetables, and water. His therapy is simple, feasible, and effective, and it can be replicated by most people who are consuming expensive hypertensive medications.

Lifestyle and Hypertension

From July 2011 to June 2012, Americans spent $8,081,000 on the top 10 hypertensive generic drugs.[394] Although some individuals are genetically predisposed to developing hypertension, most choose to take hypertensive medication even though it can be easily prevented and reversed through a healthy lifestyle change.

There are seven lifestyle changes that can lower blood pressure levels. Adopting all of the changes can lead to an 80 percent decreased risk in developing hypertension, irrespective of a family history of hypertension:[395]

1. Being overweight or obese is the major cause of hypertension. More than 75 percent of hypertension cases can be attributed to obesity. Maintaining a body mass index (BMI) of less than 25 Kg/m^2 is recommended.

2. Eating a diet high in fruits, vegetables, nuts and legumes, low-fat dairy products but low in meats, refine grains and sweets. Blood pressure levels tend to be lower in individuals who consume plant based diets,[396-398] which reduce the risk of developing coronary heart disease.[399]

3. Performing an average of 30 minutes per day of vigorous exercise.

4. Drinking no more than 1 glass of alcohol per day

5. Smoking cessation

6. Avoiding non-narcotic analgesics.

7. Taking a 400 mg of folic acid supplement daily

Reducing sodium consumption is the first dietary change most individuals make to reduce their blood pressure level. Lowering sodium intake is not as simple as cutting back on salt as it accounts for only 15 percent of sodium consumption. The majority (80 percent) of sodium comes from highly processed foods that are saturated with sodium to enhance flavor and preserve the shelf life of the food. Processed foods such as pickles, fast foods, salty snack foods, processed cheeses, bakery products, soups, soft drinks and smoked meats and sausages often contain very high levels of sodium per serving.

In addition to reducing sodium intake, increasing potassium is equally important. Potassium is an important but often overlooked mineral in preventing and treating hypertension. A study involving a group of hypertensive patients was placed on a diet low in sodium and high in potassium, and exercise. They successfully lowered their blood pressure levels by nearly 12 points within 30 days.[400]

Some potassium rich foods include: bananas, sweet potatoes, legumes, tomatoes, melons, citrus fruits, dried apricots, salmon, flounder, tuna, green leafy vegetables, poultry, and whole-grain cereals.

High Cholesterol

A high blood cholesterol level is the leading condition for which Americans consume a drug medication. Although drugs have been proven to reduce LDL (bad) cholesterol, a healthy lifestyle change can be equally effective and cost significantly less money and time.

For example, over a four week period, University of Toronto researchers compared the cholesterol-lowering ability of a plant based diet with that of a statin drug and found amazing results.[401] Participants were assigned to one of 3 groups: (1) a very-low-saturated-fat diet (control diet), (2) A combination of a very low saturated fat diet and 20 mg statin lowering medication, and (3) a diet high in plants.

At the end of the period, those who consistently ate a plant based diet reduced their LDL-cholesterol levels by an average of 29.6 percent. This improvement was comparable to the 33.53 percent reduction of those who had taken a statin drug and eaten the very low saturated fat diet. Even those individuals who did not consistently follow the diet were able to lower their cholesterol by 10 percent to 20 percent.

In addition, taking red yeast rice dietary supplement, along with a healthy diet and exercise, has proven to be effective as well. Researchers at the University of Pennsylvania and Thomas Jefferson University used red yeast rice supplements and a therapeutic lifestyle change program to successfully treat high LDL cholesterol in a small group of patients.[402] Unlike statin drugs, red yeast rice supplements did not elevate the patients' liver enzymes, which is one of a number of significant adverse effects associated with statin drugs.

Lifestyle and Heart Disease

Chronic high LDL is reportedly a precursor to developing cardiovascular disease. Cardiovascular disease is the leading cause of death in the U.S. and Mississippi. Mississippi has the highest heart disease mortality rate, 30 percent higher than the national rate. Blacks in Mississippi have the highest cardiovascular disease rate, which is likely because they tend to have multiple risk factors for the disease: obesity, hypertension, type 2 diabetes, physical inactivity, and cigarette smoking.[403]

Even though coronary heart (artery) disease is preventable and reversible through healthy lifestyle changes, Americans spend billions to pay for drug medications such as β-blockers, nitroglycerin, and calcium channel blockers, and invasive procedures like coronary angioplasty and coronary bypass surgery to treat the disease. In 2010, over 1.3 million cardiovascular procedures were performed to treat the disease.[404]

Some of the risks associated with these procedures include:

- Heart attack
- Kidney damage (caused by dye)
- Stroke
- Blood vessel damage
- Restenosis (blocking or narrowing of the artery within 6 months caused by excessive tissue growth within the treated area)

Fred Davis, 64, is a slender White male who had never had a weight problem. He was always active and ate healthy. However, he was genetically predisposed to high cholesterol.

About 8 years ago, he experienced chest pains that prompted him to see his physician. His doctor performed a heart catheter and kept him in the hospital over the weekend. On the following Monday, he was informed that he had blockage in his arteries, and a five artery bypass was performed that day.

Six weeks after the bypass surgery, his physician told him that within 10-12 years there was a 50 percent chance of his arteries re-clogging, but he could positively influence the outcome through a lifestyle change. He was advised to keep his LDL below 70 mg/dl. Fred responded by modifying his diet and exercise routine:

> I began performing 30 minutes of cardio exercise on a machine 5 – 7 days per week. I also restricted my animal protein intake, and took Vtorin, a statin to lower my bad cholesterol.

During the intervention, he never managed to lower his LDL. Achieving his health goal required additional work, and so he decided that he needed to make more significant changes. In January 2011, Fred modified his diet to eat 90 percent vegetables and fruits and 10 percent animal protein. He began taking the dietary supplement, Protandim, which has been found to prevent the formation of scar tissue in the heart. He continued his exercise routine as well.

Six months later, he was able to reduce his statin dosage by one half, but Fred was not satisfied until he was completely off the drug medication. He remained committed to his new lifestyle for the rest of the year.

He returned for his annual physical examination in January 2012, and he was ecstatic to learn that his LDL cholesterol level had dropped to 58 mg/dL; subsequently, his physician took him off the statin medication. Fred credits his lifestyle change for his good health:

> I feel so much better without animal protein in my diet. I've lost 10 pounds. I eat 3 to4 meals a day. When you're eating the right foods and physically active, you can eat as much as you want. My personal experience indicates that my circulation has improved. My sleep is also deeper

and my stamina is like it was 30 years ago. I will never go back to my old diet and lifestyle.

Reversing Coronary Heart Disease

Coronary heart disease is caused by a hardening of the coronary arteries that occurs when plaque builds up over a period of time. The risk factors for developing cardiovascular disease include: hypertension, diabetes, cholesterol levels, tobacco use, physical inactivity, poor diet, obesity, and alcohol.[405] It is estimated that 80 percent of heart disease and stroke could be prevented if individuals would make the simple but necessary lifestyle changes that could eliminate these risk factors.

One of the most respected authorities on lifestyle change therapies and coronary heart disease is Dr. Dean Ornish, a clinical researcher, physician, and author. Dr. Ornish's Program for Reversing Heart Disease is the only scientifically proven comprehensive lifestyle change program that reverses heart disease without drugs or surgery. It is now a health benefit within the Centers for Medicare and Medicaid Services' Intensive Cardiac Rehabilitation Program.[406]

The program is based on the Lifestyle Heart Trial studies that consistently demonstrated that a comprehensive lifestyle change program can reverse moderate to severe heart disease. Findings showed that patients who could walk could change and maintain a healthy lifestyle to stop the progression of coronary heart disease without consuming cholesterol drug medication.[407]

Initially, the Lifestyle Heart Trial occurred over 1 year. Patients were placed in 2 groups: (1) the intensive lifestyle change group (ILC) and (2) the usual care group (UC). The ILC group ate a low-fat vegetarian diet, avoided simple sugars, did not smoke, participated in stress management, and performed moderate exercise, but they did not consume cholesterol lowering medication. The UC group received standard medical care.

After only 1 year, the ILC group experienced a 37 percent reduction in LDL cholesterol levels and a 91 percent reduction in anginal episodes, which usually occur when the heart does not get sufficient oxygen and may cause chest pain, tightness, heaviness, or pressure. In contrast, the UC group experienced a mere 6 percent decrease in LDL cholesterol levels and an increase of 165 percent in angina episodes.

Over a five year period, a second and larger group of patients participated in the intensive lifestyle change program. They too experienced greater improved coronary health outcomes than those patients who received standard medical care.[408] The UC group experienced twice as many cardiovascular episodes than the ILC group. The UC group was more likely to have undergone coronary angioplasty and bypass surgery and/or to have been hospitalized for cardiovascular health problems than patients within the ILC group. Patients in the ILC group experienced a reduction of 72 percent angina episodes compared with a 36 percent decrease among the UC group. The UC group's reduction in angina episodes was influenced by the coronary angioplasty procedure that several patients underwent to restore their hearts.

When a person's heart is healthy, it pumps blood out of the left ventricle and the right ventricle. The left ventricle of the heart is the chamber that pumps blood to the rest of the body. It is often a factor in individuals with heart failure.

The test to determine how well the heart pumps blood is called the left ventricular ejection fraction (LVEF). LVEF is usually measured using a MRI, an echocardiogram, or CAT scan. A healthy LVEF should range between 55 percent and 70 percent. A LVEF of ≤40 percent likely means the patient has coronary heart disease. Left untreated, patients who have a LVEF ≤40 percent are likely to experience heart failure. Nevertheless, it has been proven that they too can improve the function of their heart through healthy lifestyle changes.

Researchers at the Preventive Medicine Research Institute showed that healthy lifestyle changes could reduce risk factors among coronary heart disease patients at risk of heart failure. The patients were candidates for surgery, but they opted for a lifestyle change program that consisted of diet, physical activity, stress management, and group support.[409]

At the beginning of the study, most of the patients did take medication, but during the program a significant number of them stopped taking ACE inhibitors and beta-blockers. They lowered their body weight, body fat, total cholesterol, LDL cholesterol, blood pressure, and resting heart rate. Overall, patients with a LVEF ≤40 percent experienced comparable health improvements to those patients with a LVEF ≥ 40 percent.

Even when patients choose heart surgery, they can experience worse health outcomes than those who choose to make healthy lifestyle changes. In one study, coronary heart patients who had a LVEF ≤40 percent were placed in 1 of 2 groups: the lifestyle change intervention group that adopted a low-fat diet, exercise, and stress management or 2) the surgical group.[410]

Over a 3 year period, the surgical group experienced 6 cardiac episodes compared with 1 in the lifestyle change group. Among the patients in the lifestyle change group, merely 1 died of heart disease and only 3 eventually needed to have the surgery.

These studies are further evidence that adopting a healthy lifestyle can prevent and reverse cardiovascular disease, the number 1 cause of mortality in the world. Furthermore, the benefits of making healthy lifestyle changes can be realized within a short period. Heart attacks, strokes, and related deaths can be decreased dramatically within months versus years when individuals make the necessary changes in their lives.[411]

Chapter 9

Preventing & Surviving Cancer

Even though more Americans die of heart disease, cancer remains the most terrifying chronic disease. The fear persists because cancer's high mortality rates do. Yet, while the nation remains consumed with finding an elusive cure, much could be done to prevent various cancers from ever developing. Many people are terrified of the standard toxic and extremely expensive cancer drug therapies that are often not very effective at treating most types of cancers, which are preventable.

Interestingly, the risk factors associated with common types of cancer can be reduced by making the same modest lifestyle changes that are linked to type 2 diabetes and heart disease. Cancers of the lung and bronchus, prostate, colon, and breast are all associated with modifiable behavioral factors, e.g. tobacco exposure, excessive alcohol consumption, obesity, physical inactivity, and diet, that can reduce the risk.

These risk factors may explain why cancer occurs more often and/or claims more lives among men, Blacks, and Southerners than other groups in the U.S.[412] And, helping Americans to change or eliminate these conditions may prove to be the most effective and feasible strategy in the battle against cancer.

The War on Cancer

It has been nearly 44 years since President Richard Nixon signed the *National Cancer Act* that became known as the "*war on cancer.*" Excluding the development of new and expensive drugs, very modest overall progress has occurred in the "war on cancer."

Most new drugs are developed to target specific tumor types. In many cases, these drugs are effective for merely a subset of patients with a specific tumor. The drugs often extend life for an additional few months. They are extremely expensive and contribute to the huge financial burden of treating cancer.

The cost to treat cancer is increasing at a rate of 15 percent annually,[(413)] primarily because of drug therapies. In 2007, $17.8 billion prescription drugs were sold in the U.S., and cancer drugs made up the 2nd largest category, second to cholesterol lowering drugs.[(414)] Since 2010 the average cancer drug price has cost about $10,000 per month.[(415)]

The extreme cost of treating cancer is associated with an increased rate of bankruptcies that typically occur within 2.5 years.[(416)] Elderly patients tend to have a lower chance of experiencing bankruptcy; younger patients have a much higher bankruptcy rate.

Cancer Research

Billions of federal dollars have been committed to cancer research. From 2005 to 2014, the National Cancer Institute's funding for cancer research, including cancer prevention research, averaged $4.9 billion annually, most of which was allocated to breast cancer even though more people die of lung cancer.[(417-419)]

Thanks to the billions invested in cancer prevention research, we have learned a lot about how cancer develops, metastasizes, recurs, and kills. More importantly, we have gained considerable knowledge about how some cancers can be prevented and detected early. Despite this, public health professionals have failed to integrate evidence-based cancer prevention findings into community-based intervention programs to reach those groups that have a greater risk of developing cancer.

Furthermore, society at large has failed to demand that the federal government places the same value on cancer prevention as it does on cancer research and treatment. Cancer prevention funding is trivial. From 2005 to 2014, the Centers for Disease Control and Prevention's cancer prevention funding averaged merely $329.6 million per year.[420] This amount includes funding for the most important program component of cancer prevention: the CDC's National Comprehensive Cancer Control program.

The National Comprehensive Cancer Control program is a coalition of public and private organizations throughout the nation that work together to reduce the number of people who develop and die of cancer. Several of the program's objectives include: cancer prevention through the promotion of healthy living, increasing early detection and diagnosis, and advocating for cancer control policy.

The program has the right goal, objectives, and approach needed to drastically reduce the number of people who develop and die of cancer. Unfortunately, it does not have sufficient funding to accomplish its mission, and it never has. Of the $329.6 million, the program received an average yearly amount of a meager $18.1 million.[421]

Creating Cancer Prevention Communities

The National Comprehensive Cancer Control program is likely the most significant but underutilized tactic in the "war on cancer" as it places the two most important weapons on the frontline: individuals and their communities. To win this battle, the war must be redirected to aggressively focus on cancer prevention at the individual and community level. Therefore, cancer programs must be placed within work and residential communities where individuals at risk can participate in comprehensive lifestyle change programs designed to reduce common cancer risk factors: diet, physical inactivity, alcohol, tobacco, and other controllable environmental toxins.

As early as the 1970s, evidence has shown that lifestyle is the major underlying factor in the development of most common forms of cancers: colon, breast, prostate, and lung. An individual can prevent 60 percent of cancer occurrences and about 1/3 of cancer deaths if a person merely adopts a healthy lifestyle. Researchers around the globe have generated a convincing body of data about risk factors that can influence cancer prevention, reoccurrence, and survival.

The findings strongly suggest that the most effective way to defeat cancer is to change the conditions that encourage it to develop, grow, and reoccur. Individuals must change their behavior to decrease the risk of developing cancer and increase their chance of surviving it. And, governments and employers must create communities that support anti-cancer lifestyles.

It is possible that an increase in farmers markets, organic farming, community gardens, supermarkets, community fitness centers and lifestyle intervention programs would reduce the rates of cancer incidence and death by decreasing obesity and other cancer risk factors. For instance, what if the millions of Americans who participate in annual running, walking, and cycling events to raise funds for cancer research would regularly perform these activities on the streets, sidewalks, bike lanes, and walking paths of their own communities? They would probably lower their risk of developing most cancers.

Starksville, Hattiesburg, Sumrall, and Hernando, towns located in Mississippi, are good examples of communities that are designed or being designed to reduce their residents' risk of developing cancer and other chronic conditions. These towns are developing and/or expanding bike/paths, sidewalks, community based physical activity events, farmers markets, community gardens, and tobacco control policies. Tobacco control policies are pivotal to reducing lung cancer, the number 1 cancer killer in women and men.

Tobacco Control Policies

Mississippi has one of the highest smoking rates in the U.S. The rates correlate with its high lung/bronchus cancer rate, which is the second highest in the nation. In an effort to reduce tobacco related diseases, a growing number of towns in the State have adopted smoke free legislation.

In May 2006, the town of Starkville, located in Oktibbeha County, implemented a comprehensive smoking ban in all indoor public places. The town of Hattiesburg followed suit in January 2007. Both towns have experienced a significant decline in heart attacks. Starkville residents had a 28 percent decline in heart attack hospital admissions that was almost twice the reduction of heart attacks among non-residents. The city of Hattiesburg experienced a 13.4 percent reduction in heart attack admissions compared with the 3.8 percent of nonresidents.(422)

It is possible that these policies also may have contributed to stabilizing and falling lung and bronchus rates within the counties in which the towns are located. Oktibbeha County, for example, has the lowest lung cancer incidence and mortality rates among all counties in Mississippi that have a population above 10,000.(423)

Presently, 80 municipalities in Mississippi have implemented 100 percent smoke-free ordinances,(424) but to have a greater impact on tobacco related diseases, the State must pass a statewide smoke-free ban in indoor public places, worksites, restaurants, and bars. Smoke-free legislation is supported by the overwhelming majority of Mississippians and public health professionals but not the Mississippi State Legislature.

Each year, several smoke-free bills are introduced to the Mississippi State Legislature but are defeated or not brought up for discussion. It is regrettable as such legislation would further reduce the number of Mississippians who are at risk of developing chronic diseases caused by tobacco smoke.

Overall, Mississippi's progress on key tobacco control policies is very poor, which explains why the American Lung Association assigned it a failing (F) grade in tobacco prevention, smoke-free air, cigarette tax, and tobacco cessation.(425)

Increasing tobacco cessation rates is one of the most important objectives the nation can accomplish in order to reduce the incidence of most cancer types. For example, tobacco cessation programs are responsible for the 40 percent reduction in the overall lung cancer mortality rate among men. Many more lives probably could be saved if states would pass statewide tobacco control legislation and if the Food and Drug Administration (FDA) would ban menthol brand cigarettes.

The FDA and Menthol Cigarettes

In June 2009, President Obama signed the Family Smoking Prevention and Tobacco Control Act (the Tobacco Control Act) that authorized the FDA to regulate all tobacco products within the U.S. In an effort to discourage smoking initiation, especially among youth, the FDA banned all flavored cigarettes except menthol.(426)

Menthol is an additive that produces a cooling sensation and reduces the harshness and irritation that accompanies cigarette smoke. More than 40 percent of American youth smoke menthol brand cigarettes and 30 percent of all adults, primarily Blacks. If menthol were banned from the U.S. marketplace, by 2050, over 600,000 smoking related deaths could be prevented, and over 200,000 deaths could be avoided among Blacks.(427)

Despite scientific evidence and expert recommendations to ban menthol, the FDA has chosen not to do so. Instead it charged its Tobacco Products Scientific Advisory Committee, which was composed of leading public health experts and tobacco industry representatives(428) to investigate and report on the impact of menthol brand cigarettes on the public's health.

On March 23, 2011, the Committee reported the following findings and recommendations to the FDA's Center for Tobacco Products.(429) Menthol cigarettes cause harm to public health by:

- (1) increasing the risk of smoking related diseases and (2) increasing the number of people who smoke, chiefly youth,
- Menthol cigarettes increase the probability of addiction and the degree of addiction among youth,
- It is "biologically plausible that menthol makes cigarette smoking

more addictive" and that in addition to adding flavor, menthol acts as a drug in that it changes the effects of nicotine on the smoker "by reducing the harshness of smoke and the irritation from nicotine, and may increase the likelihood of nicotine addiction in adolescents and young adults who experiment with smoking",

- The availability of menthol cigarettes reduces the likelihood that Blacks will cease smoking cigarettes,
- The tobacco industry has targeted Blacks and teens to market menthol cigarettes. Over half of all youth smoke menthol, and 80 percent of Black youth smoke menthol,
- Blacks — of all socio-economical levels, gender, age groups, and geographic locations — disproportionately smoke menthol cigarettes,
- "Taking menthol cigarettes off the market would benefit public health in the U.S."

Even with such strong and credible evidence and recommendations, Dr. Lawrence Deyton, Director of the Center for Tobacco Products of the FDA, stated the Advisory Committee's recommendation is "simply that – a committee recommendation based on its review of current, prevailing science on the topic of menthol as an ingredient in cigarettes".[(430)] He further pointed out there is no deadline or required time for the FDA to act if it chooses to do so.

Waiting for the FDA

Not satisfied with its Advisory Committee's findings and recommendations, the FDA independently conducted a thorough scientific review of menthol cigarettes and drew the following conclusions[(431)]:

1) Menthol cigarettes are not greater in toxicity than non-menthol cigarettes.

2) Adolescents and Blacks prefer menthol cigarettes because the industry targets these groups.

3) Menthol cigarettes likely increase initiation and progression to regularly cigarette smoking.

4) Menthol cigarettes probably increase dependence, and,

5) Menthol cigarettes likely decrease smokers', especially Blacks, success at quitting.

Yet, despite its own findings, the FDA has chosen not to ban menthol in cigarettes; rather, it appears to be in search of an alternative. It issued an Advance Notice of Proposed Rulemaking to allegedly "obtain additional information related to potential regulatory options it might consider, such as establishing tobacco product standards, among others". The FDA maintains that it needs more scientific information before it takes regulatory action on menthol cigarettes. It also has sought input from the general public,which predominately supports a ban. [(432)]

Meanwhile, in an effort to reduce heart disease, the FDA has prohibited the use of partially hydrogenated (artificial trans fats) oils, which are typically used within the processed food industry. FDA Commissioner Margaret A. Hamburg stated, "... reduction in the amount of trans fat in the American diet could prevent an additional 20,000 heart attacks and 7,000 deaths from heart disease each year — a critical step in the protection of Americans' health."[(433)]

Banning partially hydrogenated oils will likely help reduce heart disease in the U.S. However, banning menthol in tobacco products certainly would be much more effective in preventing heart disease, cancer, and other tobacco related diseases and deaths. Smoking remains the single leading preventable cause of disease, disability, and death.

Its critics argue that the FDA's refusal to ban menthol is due to the tobacco industry's financial influence on the executive and legislative branches of the federal government. Still others counter that the industry's impact was severely diminished by the 1998 Master Settlement Agreement. It appears that the industry's influence has drastically declined over the years, but it has not been eradicated.

The Master Settlement Agreement

In 1994, former Mississippi Attorney General Michael Moore sued thirteen tobacco companies, which produced a $4.1 billion settlement for the State. Moore's actions made Mississippi the first state to force cigarette manufacturers to reimburse it for medical costs associated with treating smoking-related illnesses. His action led to the historic Master Settlement Agreement.

The Master Settlement Agreement is a pact reached by the state Attorneys General of 46 states, five U.S. territories, Washington, DC, and five of the nation's largest tobacco companies.[(434)] The settlement awarded $10 billion annually to cover costs associated with treating smoking-related diseases and for funding tobacco prevention program. States won concessions regarding the manner in which cigarettes could be advertised and new regulatory restrictions to prevent cigarette manufacturers from directly or indirectly targeting youth.

As part of the Agreement, states are required to use a percentage of the funding to develop tobacco prevention programs, but many states are not committing sufficient funding toward this objective. A report by the Campaign for Tobacco Free Kids found that most states spend less than the amounts recommended by the Centers for Disease Control and Prevention (CDC).[(435)]

For instance, Mississippi has one of the lowest tobacco excise taxes ($.68) in the nation. Annually, it earns $261 million in tobacco revenues, but it spends $1.23 billion on tobacco related medical costs. So, it would make good fiscal sense for Mississippi to aggressively pursue tobacco prevention, but it does not. The CDC recommends that it spends $39.2 million on tobacco prevention, but it spends $9.7 million (3.7%), which was slightly higher prior to 2011.

Spending at such low levels makes it even more difficult for states to successfully push back the industry's $8.5 billion tobacco advertising and promotional campaign. During the same year of the Master Settlement Agreement, the industry spent $8.4 billion of which $87.9 million targeted Mississippians. By 2011, that amount had reached an estimated $121 million, according to the Campaign for Tobacco Free Kids. Mississippi also fails to regulate the advertising, promotion, and placement of tobacco products and forbids municipalities from doing so.

Further, the Master Settlement Agreement forbids tobacco companies from advertising their products to children through youth oriented publications, but the industry has managed to circumvent this obstacle by increasing advertising at convenience stores and gas stations where youth and young adults can purchase flavored little cigars. It also promotes menthol cigarettes in general interest magazines to which teens and young adults may be exposed in the home, especially in Black households.

Profits over People

As the FDA stated, the tobacco industry aggressively targets Blacks, but its success is partially predicated on its long relationship with the publishers of well-established Black publications. The publishers have done a great job of reporting the struggles and triumphs of Blacks in America, but they have done so while profiting from the promotion of menthol cigarettes that have contributed to the disproportionately high rates of tobacco consumption and tobacco related diseases and mortalities among Blacks.

In 1989, lung cancer prevalence and mortality rates were rising steadily among Black men and women as revenues from menthol brand cigarette advertisements climbed among well-known Black publications. During this time, the publishers of Essence, a lifestyle magazine that targets Black women, earned approximately 9 percent of its $18 million in advertisement revenue from the cigarette industry. Johnson Publishing, owner of Ebony and Jet, earned about 17 percent of its $51.4 million from cigarette advertising.[436]

Over the past 50 years, administrators of these publications have participated in advertising campaigns to target Blacks. Consequently, there has been a steady increase in menthol cigarette consumption among Blacks of various age groups. For example, from 1968 to 1975, Black smokers 16 and older increased their consumption of menthol cigarettes from 14 percent to 38 percent, respectively. Today, about 85 percent of Blacks smokers choose menthol brand cigarettes.

Menthol brand cigarette ads also appear in White magazines but at a much lower rate than in Black magazines. Of the total cigarette ads placed between 1984 and 1985, 83 percent, 59 percent, and 66 percent of menthol cigarette ads appeared in Jet, Ebony, and Essence, respectively. In contrast, 24.6 percent, 5.1 percent, and 4.9 percent of menthol cigarette advertisements appeared in *People, Time,* and *Newsweek,* respectively.[437] This pattern continued between 1998 and 2002 during which time Black publications were 9.8 times more likely than White publications to contain menthol cigarette advertisements.[438]

The trend persists despite the disproportionate number of Blacks who experience tobacco related diseases. The most prominent brands promoted in these Black publications are *Kool* and *Newport.* Newport became the best-selling menthol cigarette in 1993, according to the FDA. At least 1 full page color menthol brand *Newport* advertisement appears in nearly every issue of the magazines. In contrast, the editors reserve very little - if any- space to address tobacco related illnesses such as heart disease, respiratory illnesses, and lung cancer.

Tobacco advertising dollars were once considered important to the survival of Black publications. However, in a post-racial, consumer-driven society, these publications should be able to thrive without tobacco revenue. The industry will continue to aggressively target Blacks until the FDA bans menthol or managers of Black publications act responsibly.

The Industry Buys Influence

The U.S. Congress has failed to take any action to ban menthol. Its reluctance may be due to the industry's financial influence on some of the most liberal Democrats and conservative Republicans, who share a common interest in tobacco money.

The tobacco industry has contributed an estimated total $38 million to the U.S. Congress. Of that amount, Republicans and Democrats received 74 percent and 26 percent, respectively. President Barack Obama and Vice President Joseph Biden have received career totals of $85,694 and $24,200, respectively. U.S. senators and representatives from Mississippi have received a combined career total of nearly half a million.(439)

Poor public health policies and the absence of anti-smoking messages to counter the plethora of tobacco advertisements have effectively removed any real challenge to the tobacco industry. This void along with modest state spending on tobacco prevention programs, low to modest cigarette taxes, and a negligent state legislative body all contribute to high rates of tobacco consumption and related diseases in Mississippi. Tobacco remains one of the major risk factors that individuals can eliminate to reduce the probability of cancer developing.

Cancer Risk Factors

Cancer is defined as a buildup of clonal cells that form tumor cells, which cause disorder within the human body.(440) Cancer cells can invade multiple organs. A variety of cancer types have numerous molecular differences with different prognosis. They can be enclosed within a tumor site or metastasize, which is the cause of most cancer related deaths. As with other chronic diseases, there are various risk factors that an individual can control and change to decrease the risk of cancer developing, spreading, and re-occurring.

Although genetics can influence the risk of developing some cancers, research has demonstrated a stronger relationship between most cancers and lifestyle. An estimated 90 percent of cancer deaths in the U.S. and many developed nations are caused by unhealthy diets, tobacco and alcohol consumption, infections, and occupational exposure to toxins.

Like other chronic diseases, cancer does not develop overnight; however, it is a process that begins when an individual is exposed to a mutagen that interacts with his or her DNA and causes abnormal cell activity. It seems that the right conditions must exist for most cancers to develop, grow, and metastasize. Therefore, the following section will address modifiable risk factors that can influence the probability of most people developing common forms of cancer.

Tobacco

As mentioned earlier, tobacco consumption is the number 1 risk factor for developing most forms of cancers. In addition to lung cancer, smoking cigarettes causes acute myeloid leukemia, cancer of the bladder cancer, cervix, esophagus, kidney, voice box, lung, mouth, throat, pancreas, stomach, and the uterus. Also, it increases the risk of breast cancer and the recurrence of prostate cancer.

Smoking a pipe causes lung cancer and increases the risk of cancers of the mouth, throat, larynx, and esophagus. Smoking kreteks is associated with lung cancer and other lung diseases. Bidi use is linked to cancers of the mouth, throat, larynx, esophagus, and lung. Smokeless tobacco (snuff and chewing tobacco) causes oral cancer, esophageal cancer, and pancreatic cancer. Cigars, which contain more cancer-causing tar and releases more toxic substances, cause cancer of the oral cavity, larynx, esophagus, and lung. Cigars also linked to linked to cancer of the pancreas.(441)

The age at which a person begins smoking and the number of years the person smokes, the number of cigarettes (or other smoking instruments) smoked daily and the condition of the person's health when smoking stops determine the risk of developing and dying of some cancers.(442)

Quitting can reduce the risk of dying of various cancers. After quitting, within 10 years the risk of dying from lung cancer is reduced by 50 percent. The risk of cancer of the mouth, throat, esophagus, and bladder are reduced by half after 5 years of quitting.(443)

Alcohol

Alcohol consumption, mainly among smokers, increases the risk of developing cancer of the mouth,[444] pharynx,[445] esophagus,[446] colon,[447] larynx, liver, pancreas,[448] and breast cancer, especially hormone-sensitive breast cancer among postmenopausal women.[449-450]

One way in which alcohol may impact a woman's risk for breast cancer is through its negative effect on estrogen metabolism.[451-452] Daily consumption of alcohol is associated with higher estrogen levels that may affect breast cancer development.[453] Also, alcohol in combination with estrogen therapy may increase breast tumor growth in obese women.[454]

Alcohol may influence cancer recurrence as well. Early stage breast cancer survivors who are postmenopausal, overweight, or obese and who regularly consume alcohol have been found to have an increased risk of breast cancer recurrence and death.[455]

Breast cancer survivors who are obese, and smoke, and regularly consume alcohol may have an even greater risk of developing cancer in the other breast, known as contralateral breast cancer. For instance, a group of women who consumed ≥7 drinks per week and were current smokers were found to have a 7.2-fold increased risk of contralateral breast cancer compared with those who consumed less and had quit smoking. Obese women were found to have an elevated risk of contralateral breast cancer compared with overweight women.[456]

Alcohol can increase breast cancer risk through its negative effect on folate levels.[457-458] Increasing folate intake may offer protection among women who regularly consume alcohol.[459-461]

Bodyweight

Bodyweight is the second most important risk factor for developing most forms of chronic disease, including cancers. Like other chronic diseases, cancer rates have simultaneously increased with obesity rates. It is estimated that many cancer related deaths in the U.S. could be prevented if adults would maintain a healthy bodyweight.

Over 100 studies have found that BMI was associated with an increased incidence of a number of common and rare forms of cancers: postmenopausal breast cancer, colon, endometrial, gallbladder, pancreas, esophageal, renal, thyroid cancers, leukemia, multiple myeloma, and non-Hodgkin's lymphoma in women.[462]

Take pancreatic cancer as an example, it is a rare form of cancer with a high mortality rate, and being obese affects the risk of developing it. Men and women who are overweight or obese during early adulthood greatly increase their risk of developing pancreatic cancer and at a younger age. Also, older obese individuals who develop pancreatic cancer may be more likely to die of it.[463]

Obesity is a major factor in prostate cancer occurrence, metastasis, and survival. Obese men are at an increased risk of developing prostate cancer[464-467] and of the cancer recurring after undergoing a prostatectomy.[468]

There is a greater risk of prostate cancer metastasizing when obese patients have diabetes. Researchers at Duke University School of Medicine showed that obese men who have diabetes have a four-fold greater chance of their prostate cancer metastasizing after undergoing a radical prostatectomy.[469] Most of the obese patients were Black.

In another study, they found that a higher BMI was related to higher grade tumors and increased tumor volume among obese men undergoing radical prostatectomy. Patients whose BMI was ≥35 had almost a 40 percent larger average tumor size than normal weight prostate cancer patients. Most of the obese patients were younger and Black.[470]

Tumor grade helps determine how quickly the tumor is likely to grow and metastasize. Higher grade tumors, 3 and 4, or poorly differentiated tumors tend to grow fast and metastasize faster than tumors of a lower grade, according to the National Cancer Institute.[471] Obese women and men whose BMIs are greater than 30 mg/kg2 and 35 mg/kg2, respectively, are likely to have higher grade tumors and higher rates of cancer recurrence after treatment.

Obesity is a major determinant in cancer mortality as well. In a study that examined the cancer death rates of more than 900,000 people, obese women and men had death rates that were 62 percent and 52 percent higher, respectively, than the rates of those with normal weight.[472] These findings are comparable to other studies.[473-474]

Abdominal Obesity

BMI is typically used to determine overall obesity; however, abdominal obesity may be a more reliable predictor of cancer risk. As stated earlier, more than any part of the body, the abdominal section (waist circumference) seems to be the most dangerous place to have excess weight as it is associated with metabolic and hormonal changes that increase the risk of developing a number of chronic diseases including insulin resistance, metabolic syndrome, type 2 diabetes and various cancers.[475]

Abdominal obesity increases the risk for premenopausal and postmenopausal breast cancer, and it may place a woman at a greater risk of developing triple-negative breast cancer.[476] Triple negative breast cancer is a rare form of breast cancer that is not likely to be found on a mammogram. Its tumor lacks estrogen, progesterone, and the human epidermal growth factor receptor 2 (HER2) gene, which are common types of receptors responsible for fueling most breast cancer growth.

Triple negative breast cancer is insensitive to some of the most effective cancer therapies.[477] It is more aggressive, invasive, and deadly, and it is more likely to metastasize and reoccur. It contains p53 mutations.[478-480] The p53 gene is known as the tumor suppressor gene in that it is responsible for coding a protein that prevents the development and growth of tumors. A mutated p53 gene allows cancer tumors to develop and thrive.[481]

Triple-negative breast cancer has been shown to occur (and kill) more frequently in young Black women,[482] who also tend to have advanced cancer tumors that are of a higher grade.[483] This may be due to body weight in that Black women are more likely to be severely obese when they are diagnosed with breast cancer. They are more likely to be diagnosed with cancer at an advanced stage, to have tumor-node-metastasis (TNM) stage II or greater, and to have larger tumors.[484-485] Additionally, all women who have a high waist-to-hip ratio have an increased breast cancer risk too.[486-488]

Abdominal obesity influences a man's risk of developing cancer as well, particularly colon cancer[489] and prostate cancer. Men who have abdominal obesity may have a greater risk of prostate cancer occurring at a younger age and experiencing larger tumors.[490] Men who have large waist circumferences and waist-to-hip ratio have been shown to have a 2-fold increased risk for prostate cancer.[491]

Obesity may affect cancer through its strong association with chronic inflammation, a major factor in the development of a number of diseases: insulin resistance, type 2 diabetes, atherosclerosis, and non-alcoholic fatty liver disease,[492] dyslipidemia, cardiovascular disease, and various cancers,[493-495] such as liver, colon, breast, esophageal, and endometrium.[496]

Chronic Inflammation

Chronic inflammation occurs when the body's tissues are harmed by physical, chemical, or biological stimuli, e.g. an infection, cut, allergic reaction, toxin, and trauma. The body's inflammatory response system activates temporarily (pro-inflammatory) to eliminate harmful agents and repair the injured tissue, but sometimes the system fails to return to an anti-inflammatory state, hence chronic inflammation.[497] A chronic inflammatory state can lead to diseases such as cancer.

Research shows that more than 25 percent of all cancers are related to chronic inflammation.[498] Chronic inflammation leads to a replicated series of cell damage and the rapid reproduction of new cells that increases the number of cells dividing. This subsequently increases the risk of DNA damage that causes the promotion of malignant cells.[499] In addition to chronic inflammation, infections are a risk factor for some cancer types.

Infections

Persistent bacterial and viral infections are responsible for approximately 15 percent of the world's cancers.[500] Infections actually suppress the immune system and help initiate and promote the formation of cancerous tumors over a long period of dormancy.

Chronic Helicobacter pylori infection is linked to stomach cancer. Colon cancer is associated with chronic ulcerative colitis and Crohn's disease to inflammatory bowel diseases. Liver cancer is associated with Hepatitis C infection, and the Epstein Barr virus is related to non-Hodgkins lymphoma. Chronic Hepatitis B virus infection can cause hepatocellular carcinoma.[501]

Most cervical and anal cancers are caused by two high-risk human papillomaviruses (HPV): HPV-16 and HPV-18. These are not the same types that cause skin warts.[502] Usually the human body can eradicate high-risk HPV infections within 1-2 years, but when this does not happen, the infections can become chronic and cause normal cells to become abnormal and progress to cervical and anal cancer.

Diabetes

There appears to be a strong interaction between some cancer types, obesity, diabetes, and insulin resistance, which is associated with chronic inflammation.[503] According to researchers Kahn, Hull and Utrzschneider:[504]

> In obese individuals, adipose tissue releases increased amounts of non-esterified fatty acids, glycerol, hormones, pro-inflammatory cytokines and other factors that are involved in the development of insulin resistance.

Insulin resistance occurs when organs resist the body's attempt to transport glucose into cells for energy. Consequently, the pancreas produces too much insulin causing elevated levels of insulin in the blood. Over a period of time, this chronic condition may lead to type 2 diabetes and eventually other disorders such as cancer.

Insulin regulates the functions of body cells, and it is an essential growth factor for tissues. It can direct cells to increase quickly by increasing levels of insulin-like growth factors (IGFs).

Insulin-like growth factor is a potent protein that is involved in regulating cell proliferation, differentiation, and apoptosis (programmed cell death).[(505)] Of particular concern is IGF-1 because high levels of it are associated with an increased risk of developing cancer of the breast, colon, and prostate.[(506)] Insulin promotes the synthesis and biological activity of IGF-1,[(507)] and the two have been shown to promote cell proliferation and inhibit apoptosis.[(508-509)]

IGF-1 is necessary for growth during childhood, but it may pose a problem among adults, particularly, middle age and elderly people. A number of studies have reported that high circulating levels of IGF-1 increase the risk of common forms of cancer developing and growing, such as prostate cancer,[(510-511)] breast cancer,[(512-514)] particularly among premenopausal women, and colorectum cancer.[(515-516)] The Harvard Gazette reported:[(517)]

> In children, the hormone stimulates [IGF-1] bone growth and development of organs such as the heart, liver, and kidneys. But in older people, rapidly proliferating cells increase the opportunity for genetic mutations that may lead to cancer. And once cancer cells begin to form, IGF-1 will promote their growth as well as that of normal cells.

A synergistic relationship exists between obesity, insulin resistance, diabetes, and cancer as one condition seems to increase the risk of another occurring. This negative interaction may explain why some individuals who are obese and diabetic have an increased risk of developing various types of cancers. For example, Duke University researchers reported that pre-existing diabetes among obese prostate cancer patients was strongly associated with high-grade[(518)] disease, more secondary aggressive treatment, and a greater risk of metastasis. Metastasis was also associated with a longer duration of diabetes.[(519)]

When men and women who were diagnosed with diabetes 15 years or less were compared with those diagnosed 15 years or more. Men with a longer diabetes duration experienced higher rates of cancer of the skin, colon, and urinary tract. Women had a higher occurrence of cancer of the skin, reproductive organs, and breasts.[520]

Other studies have shown the risk of developing breast cancer is higher for women who have diabetes[521-523] but chiefly among those who are overweight/obese.[524] A diabetes diagnosis increases the risk of breast cancer patients dying as well.

Individuals who have diabetes and who later develop cancer are more likely to die [525-526] primarily from chronic diseases such as, hypertension, a heart attack,[527] and insulin resistance.[528] In one study, breast cancer patients who had type 2 diabetes experienced nearly a 40 percent increase in death during the first 5 years following the diagnosis.[529]

Also, diabetes affects the survival of breast cancer patients who have chronic hyperglycemia, a condition caused by excessive glucose circulating in the blood. It develops when the hemoglobin level A1C is ≥ 7.0 percent. Early stage breast cancer patients who have a HbA1C ≥ 6.5 percent have been shown to experience a 2.4-fold greater risk of dying from all types of diseases.[530] Most of the women were obese and Black.

Additionally, Black breast cancer patients experience a significantly higher breast cancer recurrence and progression. In one study, most Black cancer patients did not die of breast cancer but pre-existing medical conditions, primarily diabetes and hypertension. These diseases are known as *competing diseases* that complicate conventional cancer treatment.[531]

For example, hypertension, which is highest among Black women, independently accounted for a significant number of deaths among Black cancer patients according to one report.[532] Moreover, hypertension, diabetes, and high cholesterol have been found to be high among Black cancer survivors, primarily those who were obese.[533]

Glucose

High glucose levels have been implicated in the risk of developing cancer. A growing body of evidence has shown that glucose restriction may play a vital role in cancer prevention and survival. It is suggested that cancer tumor cells rely on a steady supply of glucose to form and grow. Duke University researchers demonstrated that tumor cells use glucose as a means of avoiding apoptosis by exploiting *Akt,* known as Protein Kinase B.

Akt is a key group of proteins involved in cell growth and survival,[534] and glucose metabolism.[535] According to the Duke University researchers:[536]

> In normal cells, growth factors regulate metabolism and cell survival. Removing these factors leads to loss of glucose uptake and metabolism and cell death. Cancer cells, however, maintain glucose metabolism and resist cell death, even when deprived of growth factors...

Theoretically, cancer cells metabolize glucose at higher rates than healthy cells, and cancer cells are more sensitive to glucose reduction. For instance, researchers at the University of Alabama determined that restricting glucose consumption can expand the life of normal lung cells while increasing the death of precancerous lung cells thereby preventing cancer cell proliferation and growth rate.[537]

High levels of glucose have been linked to breast cancer occurrence and survival. Pre- and post- menopausal women who have high circulating levels of glucose have been found to be at greater risk of developing breast cancer.[538] Breast cancer patients who are obese or who have high levels of fasting glucose may be more likely to die.[539]

Starving Cancer Cells

Evidence strongly suggests that diet is a major controller of glucose, insulin, and IGF-1 levels. Glucose levels can be reduced by adopting a caloric restricted diet. Insulin levels can be significantly decreased during a state of fasting, and IGF-1 levels may be reduced through protein restriction,[540] a caloric restricted diet,[541] and fasting.[542]

A high protein diet is associated with increased IGF-1 levels in men and premenopausal women. Although a high consumption of various types of protein increases IGF-1 levels, cow's milk, including skim or whole milk, has been reported to consistently increase levels among men and women.[543-544] Cow's milk naturally contains IGF-1, which has been shown to be absorbed intact.[545]

Restricting total calories may lower IGF-1 levels. A caloric restricted diet is a reduction of 10 percent – 40 percent of calories. A number of animal studies has found the diet has an anti-inflammatory effect,[546] improves t-cell function,[547] prolongs life[548] and delays some age related diseases, such as cardiovascular disease, diabetes, cancer, and brain atrophy.[549]

A popular type of caloric restricted diet is the ketogenic diet, composed of high-fat and low carbohydrate foods. Some studies have shown it to be anti-inflammatory and anti-angiogenic (prohibits the formation of new blood vessels from pre-existing vessels). It purportedly works by lowering circulating blood glucose levels, thus reducing carbohydrate energy for the tumor cells.[550]

It has been widely used to treat a variety of epileptic seizures in children and adults[551-554] and brain tumors.[555] According to researchers at John Hopkins University, it greatly exceeds medications when properly implemented.[556]

Boston College researchers have performed a number of investigations on the effects of a caloric restricted diet on malignant brain tumors. They established that a moderate (30 percent to 40 percent) caloric restricted diet significantly reduced angiogenesis (the creation of new blood vessels) and the growth of recurrent malignant brain tumors in mice.[557]

They reported that a 40 percent reduction in calories and a significant reduction in circulating IGF-1 caused considerable anti-angiogenic and proapoptotic (leads to cell death) effects in animal and human brain tumors. They concluded:[558]

> As long as brain tumor cells have access to glucose and glutamine, the disease will progress. The current standard of care provides brain tumors with access to glucose and glutamine.

Fasting

Fasting, known as short term starvation, protects normal cells by significantly reducing glucose and IGF-1 levels. It is more effective than caloric restriction because a caloric restricted diet takes months to be effective whereas fasting has a more immediate and greater effect on diminishing the levels by more than 50 percent.(559)

Researchers at the University of Southern California (USC) demonstrated the therapeutic role of fasting in cancer survival. According to their findings, fasting creates an extreme environment in which cancer cells cannot thrive. This in turn prevents cancer growth and improves the effectiveness of chemotherapy(560) It achieves this through protecting healthy cells and tissues but not cancer cells against the toxicity of chemotherapy drugs and possibly by reducing multidrug resistance.(561) Subsequently, chemo-induced side-effects are decreased and the chance of survival increased.

Fasting alone has been shown to postpone the growth of some types of cancer tumors as effective as chemotherapy drugs. It has increased chemo efficacy in treating melanoma, glioblastoma multiforme (GBM) and breast cancer cells. However, fasting and chemotherapy worked more effectively, consistently, and potently when the therapies were integrated.(562)

Fasting protects healthy cells from chemotherapy DNA damage,(563) and it improves the quality of life of cancer patients who are treated with chemotherapy.(564)

USC researchers used fasting as a complimentary therapy and showed that it significantly decreased adverse effects caused by chemotherapy. In the study, patients participated in a fast 48–140 hours prior to receiving chemotherapy and/or 5–56 hours after receiving chemotherapy. Fasting produced minor adverse effects (lightheadedness, hunger), but there was a reduction in fatigue, weakness, and gastrointestinal problems, common side effects of chemotherapy.

During the first cycle of chemotherapy, one of the breast cancer patients who participated in the fast experienced mild fatigue, dry mouth, and hiccups. She was able to work 12 hour days and pursue her usual daily activities. In contrast, when she returned to her usual diet during the 2nd and 3rd cycles of chemotherapy, she experienced moderate to severe fatigue, weakness, nausea, abdominal cramps and diarrhea. The side effects were so debilitating that she could not continue her usual schedule.

The lung cancer patient fasted for 48 hours prior and 24 hours after receiving her 6th and final cycle of chemotherapy. She experienced mild fatigue and weakness, and the chemo-induced acute toxic side effects were reduced. Her strength returned sooner, and she was able to resume physical activity.

Physical Activity

Brisk walking and other forms of physical activity reduce the risk of developing cancer through: reduction of body fat, sexual and metabolic hormones, chronic inflammation, insulin resistance, and IGF-I, and the improvement of overall immune function.

Take prostate cancer for example, physical activity has been shown to increase insulin sensitivity and decrease IGF-1 among prostate cancer patients.[565-567] In one study, prostate cancer patients who adopted an intensive exercise regimen or a low-fat diet experienced lower levels of serum insulin and IGF-1 compared with those who made no lifestyle changes. Prostate tumor cell growth was reduced in both diet and exercise groups but not the group that made no lifestyle changes. The diet and exercise group experienced a substantial increase in tumor cell death as well.[568]

Physical activity is important to a woman's overall risk for cancer development, recurrence, and survival. It confers protection against breast cancer developing throughout a woman's life.[569–573] For instance, in one study, premenopausal women who were physically active over their lifetime reduced their risk for breast cancer by 30 percent compared with those who had inactive lives.[574]

Regular physical activity may reduce breast cancer risk through its affect on hormones. It has been shown to lower estrogen and progesterone levels in premenopausal women by 19 percent and 24 percent, respectively.[575]

Physical activity is important to surviving some cancers as well. For example, breast cancer patients who are physically active have a greater likelihood of surviving it.[576] Researchers at the Moores University of California San Diego Cancer Center compared a group of sedentary early stage breast cancer patients with those who were the most physically active after cancer treatment and who sustained long term moderate to vigorous physical activity. The physically active group experienced a 53 percent reduction in breast cancer mortality and a 33 percent decrease in additional breast cancer occurrences. Survivors with poor health have been found to be obese and sedentary and to be more likely to experience cancer recurrence and death.[577]

Similar survival outcomes have been observed among prostate cancer patients. In one study, a group of men who participated in vigorous physical activity (biking, tennis, jogging, or swimming) for 3 or more hours per week experienced a 61 percent lower risk of dying from prostate cancer. Merely walking for 90 minutes or more per week reduced the risk of dying by 46 percent.[578]

Women and men can reduce their risk of developing colon cancer through regular physical activity.[579] The Memorial Sloan Kettering Cancer Center researchers found that a group of men and women who exercised 1 hour per week had a lower occurrence of colon polyps and adenomas compared with another group who exercised less or remained inactive.[580]

Performing regular light and moderate physical activity can lower the risk of developing pancreatic cancer,[581] especially among overweight individuals.[582] Individuals who have high levels of physical activity have been found to experience a 50 percent reduced risk for pancreatic cancer compared with those who have low levels.[583]

Physical activity can reduce a woman's likelihood of developing endometrial cancer as well. Among a group of women in one study, about 22 percent of endometrial cancers were prevented by regularly exercising vigorously each week.[584] Women who increased their frequency of vigorous physical activity experienced a 23 percent reduced risk of endometrial cancer in another study.[585]

There is less evidence supporting any protective benefit of physical activity against lung cancer. Some studies have produced no beneficial effect while others have. One study reported that moderate physical exercise among women who are light and heavy smokers reduced the risk of developing lung cancer,[586] and another found that medium and high levels of physical activity decreased the risk of lung cancer in both men and women.[587]

Physical activity may prevent the development of lung cancer by improving overall immune function and reducing the amount of carcinogenic agents in the respiratory system or by reducing the length of time that carcinogenic agents interact within the respiratory system.[588]

Physical activity improves physical functioning, quality of life and fatigue in cancer patients.[589] Overall, regular physical activity is one of the most important lifestyle changes an individual can make to prevent and survive most cancers, and diet is another.

Diet

There is a strong relationship between diet and the risk of developing some forms of cancer. A healthy diet reduces the risk of cancer developing primarily through maintaining a healthy body weight and lowering glucose and IGF-1 levels. In addition, nutrition provides flavonoids, antioxidants, vitamins, and minerals that are essential to maintaining an overall healthy immune system and preventing cancer.[590] According to the National Cancer Institute, approximately 35 percent of all types of cancer are linked to insufficient nutrients.(591) There is evidence that nutrition confers some degree of protection against nearly every type of cancer.

The American Institute for Cancer Research reported that the following foods provide an anti-cancer synergistic effect: apples, blueberries, berries, broccoli, Brussels sprouts, cauliflower, cherries, cranberries, dark green leafy vegetables, dry beans, peas and lentils, flaxseed, garlic, grapes and grape juice, green tea, soy, tomatoes, winter squash, and whole grains.(592)

While some foods help decrease the risk of various cancers, others have been reported to increase it. A diet high in red meat (beef, pork, lamb) and processed meat (hotdogs, sausages, links, bacon, luncheon meat, chicken nuggets and other salty, cured meats) increases an individual's risk of developing the following types of cancers: oral and pharyngeal,(593) colorectal,(594-598) prostate,(599-600) pancreatic,(601) breast,(602-605) endometrium,(606-609) esophageal,(610-612) and stomach.(613-616)

A high protein diet has been reported to promote tumor growth in breast and prostate cancers, the two most common forms of cancer in the U.S. However, a reduction of dietary protein has been shown to dramatically stop tumor growth by 56 percent and 70 percent in prostate cancer and breast cancer, respectively, by lowering serum PSA and IGF-1 levels. (617)

Breast Cancer

During each menstrual cycle, the body increases estrogen production that triggers the proliferation of cells that form the inner lining of the breast milk glands and the endometrial lining cells. From puberty to menopause, the average woman experiences hundreds of cycles of breast and endometrium cell division and programmed cell death.

Although estrogen does not directly cause DNA damage that leads to breast cancer and uterine cancer, it does speed up cell production that causes an increase in the total number of damaged (mutated) cells at risk of becoming cancerous. Many breast cancers are sensitive to estrogen, which causes cancer tumors to grow. This type of breast cancer is known as estrogen-receptor positive cancer (ER+).

ER+ cancer may be influenced by diet. Excessive estrogen production is associated with high fat diets that have been shown to increase breast cancer risk.(618-619) A reduction in dietary fat can lower estrogen levels(620) and possibly offer some protection against breast cancer developing.(621-622)

Studies have reported that premenopausal women who regularly consume red meat and high-fat dairy foods have an increased risk of developing breast cancer.(623-626) Dairy meat contains naturally occurring and synthetic growth promoting hormones. Cow's milk has a significant amount of estrogen as it comes from pregnant cows that continue to lactate through the latter half of pregnancy during which time the concentration of estrogen in the milk increases.(627) Eating low-fat dairy foods may reduce breast cancer risk among premenopausal women.(628)

Consuming less dairy fat may improve a woman's chances of surviving cancer and reduce the risk of it recurring. In a Kaiser Permanente study, women who consumed larger amounts of high fat dairy have been found to have a higher chance of breast cancer recurrence and death compared with those who consumed low fat dairy.(629)

Other foods that may protect against breast cancer include soy. The role of soy foods in breast cancer remains unclear as reports have been inconsistent. A number of studies have established that consumption of soy offers modest protection against developing breast cancer,(630-632) whereas others have found an increased risk for women who have breast cancer,(633-635) and still others have reported no relationship.

Soy foods' effect — or lack of effect — on breast cancer may be influenced by the amount and type of soy consumed and the age at which a woman begins consuming it.(636-637) Studies indicate that soy consumption at an early age offers protection against breast cancer development.(638-641)

Soy foods have been found to offer substantial protection for premenopausal Chinese women who regularly consumed soy during childhood and throughout adult life.[642] In addition to reducing the risk of breast cancer recurrence, it significantly decreased the risk of death among breast cancer survivors in China.[643-644]

Breast cancer survivors in the U.S. also have benefitted from regularly eating soy foods. In a large study of American breast cancer survivors, those who consumed levels of soy foods comparable to that of Chinese women had a lower risk of death.[645-646]

Largely, soy foods have been shown to reduce breast cancer risk among Asian women who traditionally began consuming it during childhood,[647-648] but findings regarding American women are mixed. The data suggest that American girls may need to begin consuming soy foods to receive any degree of protection against breast cancer later in life.

Walnuts may protect against breast cancer. In addition to protecting against heart disease[649] and type 2 diabetes in women,[650] walnuts may help prevent cancer at any age. Walnuts have been reported to reduce the risk of developing breast cancer[651-652] and to slow the growth of tumors in the breast,[653] prostate,[654] and colon.[655]

Pregnancy and Breastfeeding

Pregnancy and lactation permanently alter the form, structure, and molecular features of breasts that may influence breast cancer risk.[656] Pregnancy related hormonal changes cause a huge number of mammary epithelial cells to rapidly reproduce.[657] These cells line the ducts and lobes of the female breasts and produce breast milk. They also are the origin of most breast cancers.[658]

The length of breastfeeding may influence the mammary gland and subsequent risk for breast cancer. According to Dr. Nissim Silanikove, an Israeli researcher with the Agricultural Research Organization, weaning among most mammals occurs spontaneously. Natural weaning tends to happen over an ongoing period of time after the mammary gland has begun to produce significantly less milk, and the child demands less milk as well.[659]

Dr. Silanikove has suggested that abrupt or forced early weaning (between several days and 6 months) produces a "wound-like response" that may lead to an increased risk of breast cancer developing. On the other hand, natural weaning (extended breastfeeding) produces an "orderly reprogramming" of the mammary gland tissue that may actually protect it against breast cancer.

Weaning causes the mammary gland to return to its pre-pregnancy state until the next pregnancy. It also activates the removal of residual milk and milk-producing epithelial cells that are no longer needed through apoptosis (programmed cell death), which occurs in all multicellular animals.(660-662) Christine Watson, Professor of Pathology at Cambridge University, wrote:(663)

> Cell death is essential during embryonic development for the formation and development of organs and tissue sculpting and to maintain cellular homeostasis in adult organisms. Importantly, while excessive apoptosis can lead to degenerative diseases, insufficient apoptosis can result in cancer.

Weaning may help explain why breast cancer rates tend to be lower among women who have more than 1 child and who breastfeed each child for extended periods of time. The World Health Organization recommends that babies be exclusively breastfed for the first 6 months of life and that breastfeeding continues along with complimentary solids from 6 months to 2 years or longer.(664) Many international studies have concluded that breastfeeding for extended periods of time reduce the risk of developing some subtypes of premenopausal cancer.(665-674)

An analysis of over 80 percent of data from 30 nations showed that women who had more births and a much longer lifetime breastfeeding period experienced lower rates of breast cancer. The risk for local and metastasized breast cancer decreased for each birth and year of breastfeeding. Women who breast-fed for longer periods of time were less likely to reside in the U.S. and other rich nations. Women in rich nations had a lifetime breastfeeding period of 8.7 months compared with women in rural developing nations of Africa and Asia who had 29.2 months breastfeeding experience.[675]

Current and available data show that women in East and Southern Africa and South Asia have the highest breastfeeding rates, 20-23 months, in the world.[676-677] In contrast, women in Europe and North America have the lowest extended breastfeeding rates and highest breast cancer rates in the world. In fact, Europe's rate of new breast cancer cases is double that of Africa.[679]

Although breast cancer occurs less often in poor nations, there is an upward trend in incidence. Poor nations, like India, are expected to experience 70 percent of the world's cancer cases by 2020. One factor driving the increase is rapid urbanization that has led to the adoption of modern and unhealthy lifestyles. For instance, urban Indian women have assumed a lifestyle akin to women in the West. They have less children and shorter periods of breastfeeding than women who live in rural communities of India. Also, they have adopted a western diet and have higher rates of alcohol consumption and obesity.[680]

Prostate Cancer

Like breasts, the prostate gland contains specific estrogen receptors. An increase in circulating estrogen levels increases a man's risk of prostate cancer developing and progressing.[681-682] Over a male's lifetime, he is exposed to estrogen in several ways. During the third trimester of pregnancy the male fetus is exposed to high levels of estrogen in utero. He also is exposed to estrogen as he ages[683] and through dietary fat.

In general, men who consume high levels of animal fat, specifically red meat, may have an increased risk of developing localized prostate cancer[684-685] and advanced prostate cancer.[686] Consuming high levels of meat, especially process meats, and dairy may increase the risk for non-advanced prostate cancer,[687] and metastatic prostate cancer too.[688]

Among American men, Black men have a greater prostate cancer risk, but it may be because of their high intake of animal fat, not race. When compared with White men, all types of red meat were linked to a 2-fold increased risk of prostate cancer among Black men, according to a large study by the National Cancer Institute. The greatest risk was associated with cooked processed meats, chiefly bacon and sausage, which Black men consumed about 3 times more than White men.(689)

These findings are comparable with studies that showed a greater consumption of foods high in animal fat was associated with an increase in prostate cancer among Black men and advanced prostate cancer among both Black men and White men. Once again, Black men consumed more animal fat and protein. Black men who had higher levels of education and income were too at an increased risk of developing prostate cancer.(690)

Meat Preparation

The risk of eating meat may be attributed to how it is prepared, especially when it is cooked at high temperatures, specifically above 300°F, e.g. smoking, frying or grilling over an open flame. When muscle meats are cooked at high temperatures it causes the formation of chemicals known as heterocyclic amines (HCA) and polycyclic aromatic hydrocarbons (PAH).(691)

HCAs and PAHs cause changes in DNA that increase cancer risk. For instance, red meats and processed meats cooked well-done, e.g. grilled or barbequed, have been shown to produce HCA and PAH that have been linked to advanced prostate cancer.(692-695) In an animal study, mice that consumed a diet high in HCAs developed cancer of the colon, breast, prostate, lung, liver, and skin.(696) Those mice that consumed PAHs developed leukemia, lung cancer, and gastrointestinal tract cancer.(697)

In a human study, USC researchers examined the meat intake and cooking methods of Black men and White men who had been diagnosed with aggressive prostate cancer. Most were college graduates.(698)

Men who had a higher intake of beef, hamburger, and chicken that was primarily grilled, barbequed, cooked well, or very well-done experienced a much greater risk of developing aggressive prostate cancer. On the other hand, men who consumed rare or medium cooked red meat were less likely to experience aggressive prostate cancer. Ground meat that was not grilled or barbecued did not increase the risk of aggressive prostate cancer. Aggressive prostate cancer was associated with consumption of higher fat lunch meats and liver.

A study funded by the National Cancer Institute examined the relationship between HCA levels in meat and prostate cancer.(699) It concluded that the risk of developing localized prostate cancer was about 20 percent higher among those Black men who consumed more red meats that were cooked at high temperatures compared with those who consumed meat cooked at lower temperatures. Those who consumed high levels of steak and hamburgers experienced a 30 percent increased risk of prostate cancer. These findings strongly suggest that diet, not race or income, is a risk factor in the disproportionately high prevalence of prostate cancer among Black men.

Dairy and Beverages

Meat and dairy are associated with an increased risk of prostate cancer metastasizing. A high consumption of beef, processed meats, bacon, pork, lamb, and dairy may increase the probability of prostate cancer spreading.(700) Numerous studies have reported that a high consumption of dairy foods, specifically milk, can significantly increase the risk of prostate cancer developing,(701-705) progressing, or spreading.(706-709) Consuming whole milk increases the risk of dying from prostate cancer,(710-711) but non-dairy calcium sources may reduce the risk.(712)

Organic cow's milk was found to substantially stimulate prostate cancer cells, but almond milk suppressed it.(713) Soy foods may decrease the risk of prostate cancer developing(714-716) and the high risk of it spreading outside of the prostate gland.(717-718)

Men may find some protection against prostate cancer by drinking pomegranate juice. It has been shown to effectively treat a number of urological disorders, such as benign prostatic hyperplasia,[719] erectile dysfunction,[720] and prostate cancer.[721] Researchers at the University of California at Los Angeles reported that daily consumption of 8 oz of pomegranate juice significantly extended PSA doubling time, decreased cell proliferation, and increased cancer cell death in men whose PSA progressed following radiation or surgery.[722] It has prevented cell and tumor growth in highly aggressive prostate cancer in several studies.[723-725]

Coffee drinkers may have a reduced risk of prostate cancer, according to several studies. Men who drank coffee experienced a reduced risk of localized[726-728] aggressive and lethal forms of cancer.[729-730] Those who consumed the most coffee (regular or decaffeinated) experienced a 50 percent reduced risk of lethal prostate cancer.

Colon Cancer

Individuals who regularly eat red meats, processed meats, and well-done meats may have a higher risk of experiencing colon cancer. However, dairy milk, calcium, and garlic may offer some protection.[731-736]

The high intake of these meats may be a factor in the high rates of colon cancer among Blacks. Blacks have the highest rates of colon cancer incidence and mortality. They have a higher consumption of HCAs but lower levels of vitamin D,[737] which reportedly protects against colorectal cancer.[738-741]

Pancreatic Cancer

Individuals who have a diet high in sugar may have an increased risk for pancreatic cancer.[742] Men who regularly consume candy[743] and women who frequently consume sugar sweetened beverages[744-746] were found to have an increased risk. The risk is significantly increased among women who have insulin resistance.[747-748] Foods containing folate may protect against pancreatic cancer.[749]

Oral Cancer

Eating non-starchy vegetables, e.g. broccoli, Brussels sprouts, greens, and fruits, may protect against cancers of the mouth, pharynx, and larynx and esophagus.[750]

Stomach Cancer

Non-starchy and allium vegetables, e.g. garlic and onions, and fruits, may protect against stomach cancer.[751]

Lung Cancer

In general, fruits and vegetables offer protection against lung cancer.[752] Smokers consume fewer vegetables and fruits compared with former smokers and those who have never smoked. A lower risk of lung cancer was associated with elevated serum levels of $B_{6,}$ methionine, and folate, according to a very large study by the European Prospective Investigation into Cancer and Nutrition.

Healthy dietary sources of B_6 include chickpeas, salmon, banana, nuts, marinara sauce, bulgur, squash, spinach, raisins, and watermelon. Sources of methionine include: seaweed, spirulina, seeds, sesame flour, and soy protein.[753]

There is no guarantee that adopting a healthy lifestyle will prevent the development, progression, recurrence or survival of most cancers, but it can prevent excessive body weight, which leads to insulin resistance and other conditions that increases the risk of developing or dying of common forms of cancer.

Complementary and Alternative Medicines

Many cancer patients consume some form of complementary and alternative medicine (CAM), particularly dietary supplements, to improve the efficacy of standard treatment. The Mayo Foundation and Mayo Clinic College of Medicine reported that about 90 percent of its cancer patients simultaneously used CAM while receiving chemotherapeutic therapy.[754] An earlier study reported over 83 percent of North American cancer patients, particularly those with advanced disease, used CAM.[755]

The following is a brief overview of some complimentary and alternative medicines that have been shown to provide chemopreventive benefits and others that have lessened the adverse side effects of standard therapies such as chemotherapy and radiation.

Vitamin D

Researchers showed that vitamin D reduced the risk of overall mortality,[756] and lowered the risk of developing and dying of cancer of the colon, prostate, ovarian, and breast.[757]

A vitamin D deficiency also increased the risk of developing breast cancer,[758] especially estrogen-negative breast cancer, which occurs more often among Black women.[759] Deficiency may increase the risk for early and aggressive prostate cancer.[760] Most Americans are deficient in vitamin D, but Black women have the highest deficiency level.[761-762]

A healthy amount of sun exposure is the best way to get vitamin D. Dark pigmentation and all day use of sun screen protection are leading causes of vitamin D deficiency. The high levels of melanin absorbs the UV photons in dark skinned people.[763] Sun screen products typically used among pale and light skinned people block the sun's ability to photosynthesize vitamin D in the skin.[764-765]

The National Academy of Sciences recommends the following daily intake: 1 – 50 years of age, 200 IU; 51 – 70 years, 400 IU per day, and 71 years and over, 600 IU. Taking 2000 IU per day is the safe upper limit, but vitamin D becomes toxic when regular consumption exceeds 10,000 IU per day.[766]

Fish Oil

Fish oil has been reported to increase vitamin D levels.[767] Fish oil has reduced the risk of developing ductal breast cancer,[768] breast cancer metastasis to the bone,[769] and advanced prostate cancer.[770]

Supplementing chemotherapy with fish oil oil has been found to increase its effectiveness by 2-fold in patients with advanced non-small lung cancer. Patients who received fish oil in combination with chemotherapy experienced a lower cancer progression rate and a higher 1 year survival rate than those patients who received only standard care. [(771)]

Patients who consumed fish oil along with chemotherapy experienced slow tumor growth and lower metastatic load.[(772)] Another study reported that fish oil produced an increase in body weight and prevented the decrease of neutrophils, white blood cells that fight infections.[(773)]

Flaxseed

Flaxseed, an omega-3 fatty acid, has been shown to hinder breast cancer growth and metastasis in estrogen receptor negative breast cancer,[(774)] reduce tumor growth in estrogen receptor positive breast cancer, prevent the formation of new blood vessels,[(775)] and prevent metastasis after surgical excision of the breast tumor.[(776)] Flaxseed oil has been shown to reduce the growth of estrogen receptor-positive breast tumors treated with Tamoxifen.[(777)] It has reduced prostate tumor proliferation before surgery[(778)] and the growth of prostate cancer cells.[(779)]

Curcumin

Curcumin, an ingredient in turmeric, has been found to have chemopreventive effects. A number of studies have reported that it causes an apoptotic effect in various types of cancer cells, such as gastric and colon cancer cells, [(780)], stomach and skin tumors, [(781)] prostate cancer cells, [(782)] and lung cancer cells.[(783)]

Folate

Women who frequently consume alcohol may reduce their cancer risk by increasing their folate acid intake. Folate acid may protect against oral and pharyngeal cancer[(784)] and breast cancer[(785-788)] According to Drs. Hillman and Steinberg, alcohol has an adverse effect on folate. They wrote: [(789)]

> Alcohol interferes with several aspects of normal folate transport and metabolism including dietary intake, intestinal absorption, transport to tissues, storage, and release by liver, thereby disrupting folate supply to tissues.

Glutamine

Glutamine is a non-essential amino acid. Cancer tumors cause glutamine levels to significantly decrease.(790) Cancer patients who undergo chemotherapy may benefit from taking glutamine supplements during and after chemotherapy. It has been found to significantly reduce the duration and severity of stomatitis (inflammation and soreness of the mouth) caused by chemotherapy.(791) It has reduced the duration of mouth pain and the restriction of solid foods.(792)

Another study showed that glutamine reduced the severity of peripheral neuropathy associated with high-dose chemotherapy among stage 4 breast cancer patients(793) and colorectal cancer patients.(794) Cancer patients who received glutamine have been reported to experience significantly less weakness, less loss of vibratory sensation, and less toe numbness compared with those who did not consume the supplement.(795)

Astaxanthin

Astaxanthin is an antioxidant that naturally occurs in algae, fungi, crustaceans, and fish. In animal studies, it caused programmed cell death in liver cancer cells,(796) suppressed colitis-related colon cancer,(797) cell death in colon cancer,(798) delayed,(799) suppressed tumor growth,(800-801) and inhibited tumor proliferation and(802-803) cancer metastasis.(804) A combination of astaxanthin and saw palmetto decreased the growth of human prostate cancer cells.(805)

Astragalus

When combined with chemotherapy, astragalus increased the efficacy of chemotherapy that led to a reduction in the risk of death and improved tumor response among patients with non-small-cell lung cancer.[806] When a group of cancer patients received chemotherapy and astragalus, their survival rate improved and the tumor response increased.[807]

Protandim®

Protandim® has been found to suppress skin cancer tumors.[808-809] In one study, mice that were fed Protandim experienced a substantial reduction in skin tumor incidence and the number of tumors.

Mistletoe Extracts

Mistletoe extracts used in combination with chemotherapy may reduce chemo's toxic adverse effects. Early stage breast cancer patients who received Viscum album L, a mistletoe extract, during chemotherapy cycles experienced an increase in quality of life. The extract may prevent patients from delaying or stopping chemotherapy cycles.[810]

Gastric cancer patients who received the extract in conjunction with chemotherapy experienced a decrease in diarrhea and an increase in leukocyte- and eosinophil counts, white blood cells.[811] Mistletoe extracts have been shown to delay tumor growth and[812] cell death[813] in glioblastoma.

Raw Garlic

A number of small studies have reported that garlic has anti-cancer effects including apoptosis, anti-proliferation and an increase in natural-killer cell activity in various cancers: stomach,[814-815] endometrial,[816] colon,[817] prostate,[818-819] oral,[820] and breast.[821-822]

Grapeseed Extract

Grapeseed extract supplement may reduce the risk of developing prostate cancer,[823] inhibit prostate cancer growth, and progression.[824-826] It has been reported to cause cell death.[827-829]

Green Tea

Epigallocathechin-3 gallate (EGCG), a naturally occurring ingredient found in green tea, inhibits urokinase (uPA). uPA is a proteolytic enzyme that cancer cells use to invade healthy cells and metastasize. Preventing uPA has been shown to reduce tumor size and cause complete remission.[830] Green tea been has been reported to have anti-tumor effects on breast cancer.[831-833] It was found to prevent breast cancer from developing and recurring.[834]

Oral Enzymes

Oral enzyme preparation may improve the outcome of colorectal cancer patients who undergo standard cancer therapies. According to a Poland study, patients who received oral enzymes experienced a reduction in adverse effects caused by chemotherapy and radiotherapy. Although it did not reduce the number of deaths, it did extend survival time.[835]

German researchers reported that breast cancer patients who received standard cancer therapies supplemented with oral enzymes experienced significantly less adverse effects, such as: gastrointestinal symptoms, mental symptoms, dyspnoea, headache, tumor pain, cachexia, skin disorders, infections, and side effects. Rates of recurrence and metastasis decreased as well.[836]

Researchers at University of Brastislava in Slovak Republic found significant benefits in combining oral enzyme preparation with standard chemotherapy over a six month period. Patients with multiple myeloma stages I-III experienced substantial increases in overall response rates, longer duration of remission and survival.[837]

Probiotics

A study in Finland showed that a daily dosage of lactobacillus supplements can reduce chemo-induced adverse effects. Colorectal cancer patients whose treatment was supplemented with lactobacillus experienced less diarrhea, abdominal discomfort, bowel toxicity, and chemotherapy-dose reductions.[838] Other studies have found it to reduce diarrhea[839] and improve bowel functions caused by radiotherapy.[840]

Homeopathy

Cancer patients may find some homeopathic medicines useful in preventing and treating two common negative side-effects caused by chemotherapy and radiation. *Topical calendula,* known as marigold, was found to be superior to *Trolamine,* a drug medication, in treating acute dermatitis caused by radiation therapy.[841]

Fluoric acid, a homeopathic medicine, was successfully used to treat severe itching caused by radiation in breast cancer patients.[842]

Homeopathy was reported to significantly improve "estrogen withdrawal" symptoms including anxiety, depression, and quality of life among breast cancer patients.[843]

Traumeel S, a homeopathic medicated mouthwash, was significantly effective at reducing the severity and duration of inflamed and sore mouths caused by chemotherapy among children who received stem cell transplants.[844]

Acupuncture

Acupuncture is a traditional Chinese therapy that involves the insertion of extremely thin needles through the skin at strategic points on the body. It is typically used to treat pain (low back, menstrual, labor, dental pain, osteoarthritis, tennis elbow and fibromyalgia).

The therapy has been shown to be effective in addressing a number of health issues among breast cancer patients that are caused by cancer and chemotherapy. Some findings include: preventing hot flashes and sleep disturbances among postmenopausal breast cancer survivors,[845] alleviating joint pain and stiffness caused by aromatase inhibitor therapy in postmenopausal breast cancer patients[846] and early stage breast cancer patients,[847] increasing rates of salivary flow among patients with head and neck cancer who received radiation therapy,[848-850] decreasing cancer-induced depression and improving sleep quality,[851] managing chemotherapy-induced peripheral neuropathy,[852-855] reducing chemotherapy-induced vomiting and nausea,[856] increasing levels of alertness during chemotherapy, and reducing nausea and vomiting among pediatric cancer patients.[857]

Hyperthermia

The National Cancer Institute defines hyperthermia as "a type of cancer treatment in which body tissue is exposed to high temperatures (up to 113°F) to damage and kill cancer cells".[858] Typically, hyperthermia is used in combination with chemotherapy and radiotherapy. It has been effective in reducing the size of tumors in various forms of cancer, but not all studies have shown an increase in survival.[859-861]

A study involving patients with various forms of cancer received hyperthermia alone or in combination with other therapies. Those who received it alone experienced complete response rates ranging from 50 percent to 75 percent. The complete response rates endured from 1 month to 2 years. When hyperthermia was combined with radiotherapy the complete response rates were found to be higher.[862] Hyperthermia has a duration response rate of 6 weeks on average.[863]

Massage Therapy

Massage therapy may improve the quality of life of cancer patients. A group of cancer patients who received 30 minutes of massage therapy reported feeling more relaxation, less anxiety, and a reduced level of pain perception.[864] Advanced cancer patients realized an improvement in pain and sleep.[865] Pediatric cancer patients have benefitted from massage therapy as well.[866] Care givers of cancer patients have experienced reductions in anxiety, fatigue, and depression.[867]

Reflexology

Advanced breast cancer patients who received reflexology (foot manipulation) reported experiencing a decrease in the severity of dyspnea (breathing difficulty).[868] Breast and lung cancer patients who received 30 minutes of foot reflexology experienced a significant decrease in anxiety and pain,[869] including cancer patients whose partners performed the foot reflexology.[870]

Yoga

Among breast cancer patients, yoga has been reported to significantly reduce stress, anxiety, and depression; to moderately reduce fatigue; to increase overall quality of life, emotional, and social functioning,[871] and improve balance and flexibility.[872] Patients who participated in yoga breathing technique exercises experienced an improvement in sleep, anxiety, and mental quality of life.[873]

Selenium

Selenium is an essential trace element administered orally or intravenously to reduce adverse effects caused by chemotherapy and radiotherapy. It has improved the quality of life of patients with secondary head and neck lymphedema caused by radiotherapy or in combination with surgery.[874] Selenium has notably reduced postoperative lymphedema after oral tumor surgery.[875] It has increased the effectiveness of combined physical decongestion therapy and heat tolerance among post-mastectomy patients with secondary lymphedema of the arm.[876]

Final Word on Cancer Prevention

The most effective yet underutilized weapon in the "war on cancer" is the public. Lay people can play a much greater role in the battle to reduce cancer incidence and mortality rates than merely donating money to cancer research. They can start by changing unhealthy behaviors that increase their risk of developing various cancers. Furthermore, they can collectively work with their local and state governments and employers to transform their neighborhoods and worksites into communities that support anti-cancer lifestyles.

Chapter 10

Maintaining Bone Health

On a beautiful sunny and dry afternoon, I went on my usual bike ride within my neighborhood, a community that has no bike lanes, biking/walking paths and nearly no sidewalks. Typically, my son and I ride together, but on this day I rode alone. On my route home, I waited in front of the turning lane at a major intersection for the traffic light to change to green. I stood up and began to pedal, and that is the last thing I recall about that day. The next day I awoke in the University of Mississippi Medical Center (UMMC) where I had undergone emergency surgery.

According to eyewitness accounts and the police report, a 28 year old woman, who was uninsured, unemployed, and whose drivers license was suspended drove her SUV through the red light at 40 mph and struck me, knocking me about 10 feet off my bike. The impact completely shattered my right femur, but my brain was intact, thanks to my helmet.

The driver told the police that she did not see me because she was talking on the cell phone. In other words, she was distracted. Her reckless behavior added one more victim to the list of cyclists who have been struck by distracted and mentally impaired cell phone drivers. Like other incidences in Mississippi where cyclists have been severely injured or killed, she was fined a misdemeanor and allowed her to drive away with another opportunity to injure or kill someone.

Driving Under the Influence

When the driver's brain becomes engaged in a cell phone conversation she morphs into a person who is impaired as she is distracted from the act of driving, the environment, and everyone and thing within it. She is no longer fully cognizant or able to adequately and timely respond to all the various players and occurrences that take place within the environment.

The woman who nearly killed me revealed that she had not seen me even though it was a clear, sunny, and dry day. And I was wearing a brightly colored top and blue helmet. My red bike was situated in front of the traffic within the center of the intersection. Although she did not see me, all of the other drivers within the intersection did, but they were not distracted by a cell phone conversation.

Clearly, the cell phone driver is another dangerous element on the road and must be handled accordingly. In an effort to reduce injuries and deaths associated with cell phone drivers, a number of states have passed laws banning hand-held cell phones. However, these types of accidents do not occur because the driver is holding the steering wheel with one hand while gripping the cell phone with the other. Regardless of the type of phone in use, the driver is distracted because her brain is engaged in a phone conversation. Consequently, the hands-free and hand-held cell phones are equally dangerous as both have the same adverse effects on the driver's brain, according to research findings.

Researchers at the University of Utah have performed numerous studies on the dangers of driving while using cell phones. In one study, they showed that unlike cell phone conversations, when a driver communicates with a passenger the focus of the conversation tends to adapt to the circumstances on the road, such as a vehicle suddenly stopping or slowing in front of the car.[877] They reported the following findings [878-883]:

- When drivers were conversing on either a hand-held or hands-free cell phone, their braking reactions were delayed. They were involved in more traffic accidents than when they were not conversing on a cell phone.

- When drivers were talking on both types of phones they missed twice as many simulated traffic signals as when they were not. They took longer to react to traffic signals they missed.
- The abilities of both young and older drivers were adversely affected by talking on cell phones. Compared with no cell phone conversations, when drivers talked on cell phones their reactions were 18 percent slower and their following distance was 12 percent greater. They took 17 percent longer to recover the speed that was lost following braking, and they experienced a twofold increase in the number of rear-end collisions.
- Drivers who talked on a hands-free cell phone looked directly at objects in their surroundings but were less likely to develop long lasting memory of those objects such as recognizing billboards. They developed impaired reactions to vehicles braking in front of them.

These findings prove the issue is not driving while holding a cell phone, but, it is driving while talking on any type of cell phone. It may explain why state laws banning the hand-held phone have not significantly reduced cell phone related accidents. Drivers have simply switched to a hands-free cell-phone, but they remain distracted and at risk of crashing into another vehicle, pedestrian, or cyclist. This is why it is so important for the vulnerable cyclist, especially child, to wear a helmet to prevent traumatic brain injuries.

Traumatic Brain Injuries

Medical experts were shocked that I survived the accident and I did so without losing my leg, experiencing paralysis or a severe traumatic brain injury. I credit my helmet for my survival, and if more cyclists would wear helmets many deaths would likely be prevented. About 70 percent of all fatal bicycle crashes involve head injuries, but only 20 percent – 25 percent of all bicyclists wear bicycle helmets.

Bicycle helmets are the single most effective method to protect the brain against injuries during a crash.[884] The hard shell "protects the skull at point of impact and absorbs, redistributes, and releases energy rapidly," and the cushioning "reduces head impact acceleration and thus force on brain," according to Eric Blackman of the University of Rochester.[885] Although the helmet can protect the brain, a shattered femur is another matter.

Bone Health

The UMMC resident surgeon implanted a rod and numerous screws to provide support while the bone regenerated. I will never forget his declaration that I would live with the hardware for the rest of my life. I rejected that prognosis as I believed that I would fully heal with proper time, physical therapy, and bone nutrients, such as calcium.

Calcium

Like most Americans, I had assumed that consuming a lot of calcium based foods and dietary supplements would help restore my femur. Americans are encouraged to regularly drink dairy milk for bone health. This is primarily due to the ubiquitous dairy milk ads and U.S. subsidies. The dairy industry has received $5.3 billion over the past 18 years, making dairy the 9th largest recipient of farm subsidies.[886]

Dairy remains an important staple in the American diet because it is a major source of calcium. Calcium is necessary for building and strengthening bones, but the amount and type of calcium required is questionable. A number of large and long studies have investigated the relationship between dairy, calcium, and bone health. The findings will likely be disquieting for many Americans.

Take the 12 year study that followed over 77,000 middle aged women, who were registered nurses and resided in eleven states. Neither a diet high in calcium nor dairy milk protected them against hip or forearm fractures. In addition, women who consumed higher amounts of dairy based calcium experienced substantially increased risks of a hip fracture, but those who consumed the same levels of calcium from non-dairy foods did not. Women who had a higher protein intake had a greater risk of experiencing a forearm fracture.(887)

A similar study involved over 51,000 middle aged and elderly male healthcare professionals who were followed for an 8-year period. Men who consumed dairy or non-dairy calcium sources, including calcium supplements, were not protected against forearm or hip fractures.(888)

A Swedish study that followed 65,000 women, who consumed high levels of dairy, found that it did not protect them against hip fractures. It also reported that deficiencies in iron, magnesium, and vitamin C were independent risk factors for hip fractures.(889)

A 15 year study of over 1400 elderly women and men in Britain showed that a decrease in physical activity, not dietary calcium, increased their risk of experiencing a hip fracture.(890)

So, it appears that consuming high levels of calcium, particularly from dairy milk, which happens to be the top food allergen in children,(891) may not be vital to bone health after all. In fact, nations that have the highest consumption rates of dairy milk tend to have the highest osteoporosis rates as well.(892-893)

Additionally, there are alternative non-dairy calcium sources: Sardines, collard greens, Black-eyed peas, salmon, tofu, hazelnuts, parsley, turnip greens, Brazil nuts, salmon, sun flower seeds, canned baked beans, watercress, garbanzo beans, Black beans, pinto beans, pistachios, kale greens, sesame seeds, and walnuts.

In addition to calcium, there are other over-looked nutrients that are important to building and maintaining bone health: vitamin D, vitamin K, potassium, and magnesium. The following is an overview of each nutrient and its dietary sources.

Vitamin D

Vitamin D is essential to bone health, and the body needs sufficient levels of vitamin D to adequately absorb calcium. As stated earlier, many Americans are deficient in vitamin D. Vitamin D deficiency can cause bones to become thin or brittle, and a loss of muscle strength can occur, all of which increases the chance of falling and experiencing hip fractures. Daily consumption of vitamin D- not milk or a high calcium diet- was shown to reduce the risk of lower hip fractures by 37 percent among a very large group of postmenopausal women.[(894)]

Vitamin K

Vitamin K regulates calcium in the blood, prevents the creation of materials that can break down bone, and helps to build bone. Individuals who consume lower levels of vitamin K foods have a greater risk of experiencing hip fractures.[(895-897)] Vitamin K food sources include: kale, spinach, collard greens, Swiss chard, turnip greens, mustard greens, Brussels sprouts, parsley, romaine lettuce, broccoli, thyme, romaine lettuce, sage, oregano, cabbage, celery, sea vegetables, cucumber, leeks, cauliflower, tomatoes, and blueberries.

Potassium and Magnesium

Potassium and magnesium are important to bone health too. Higher consumption of both nutrients from vegetables and fruits has been reported to improve bone mineral density in the hips of elderly men and women.[(898-900)]

Potassium sources include: banana, apricots, cantaloupe, honeydew, oranges, grapefruit, prunes, celery, Swiss chard, spinach, artichoke, broccoli, tomatoes, lima beans, almonds and sunflower seeds.

Magnesium food sources include: wheat bran, almonds, spinach, raisins, cashews, soybeans, wheat germ, mix nuts, bran flakes, shredded wheat cereal, and dry roasted peanuts, peanut butter, potato skins, black eye peas, pinto beans, brown rice, lentils, and kidney beans.

Vitamin A

Adequate levels of vitamin A are necessary for vision, normal growth, and development of body tissues. High levels of vitamin A are associated with osteoporosis according to several studies. In one study, the risk of experiencing a hip fracture was nearly doubled among women who were not taking hormonal therapy but consumed vitamin A levels of 2000 µg/d or more compared with those whose intakes were less than 500µg/d. Supplements and multivitamins were the primary source of vitamin A. On the other hand, women who consumed beta carotene (liver and carrots) did not experience an increased risk of hip fractures.(901)

Excessive consumption of vitamin A derived from cod liver oil, fortified dairy milk, and dairy products has been shown to reduce bone mineral density and increase the risk of experiencing a hip fracture.(902)

Physical Activity

More than any nutrient, physical activity seems to provide more protection against bone fractures as we age. Physical activity is important for bone mass throughout the lifespan as it continually stimulates increases in bone diameter that decreases the risk of fractures by neutralizing the thinning of bones and bone porosity.(903)

Penn State University researchers have produced a number of interesting findings that show the positive role of exercise in bone health among female adolescents. A 10-year study found that **only** exercising during adolescence significantly increased bone mineral density and bone bending strength, but not daily consumption of calcium.(904)

They reported that exercise and physical fitness have a favorable effect on bone mineral density, the femoral neck and shaft in young adult women, but daily consumption of calcium had little and possibly no effect in female adolescents.(905) The amount of physical activity that a teen accumulates between 12 and 18 years of age is associated with a significant increase in hip bone mineral density at age 18 year; however, taking calcium on a daily basis had no effect.(906)

Regenerated

My journey to full recovery was long and painful. I increased my consumption of bone building foods and consumed a vitamin D supplement but not calcium. My diet remained free of dairy.

Recovery required two surgeries and two years of physical therapy for my femur to completely regenerate so I could be physically active again. I attribute my healing to physical therapy and the outstanding staff, particularly Dr. Ruth Burgess, at UMMC. In addition to helping me to walk again, the physical therapists helped me to build an overall stronger and healthier body.

Making Roads Safer

Since my accident, at least 96 pedestrians and 11 bicyclists have been killed by motor vehicles on the roads and streets of Mississippi.[907] Over 90 percent of the accidents occurred during dry weather conditions and light traffic. The degree to which cell phones or alcohol were involved is unknown as the State does not require the investigating officer to perform a blood alcohol content (BAC) test or document cell phone usage.

Safety is a major reason why many Americans do not walk and cycle. Nearly 40 percent of communities in the U.S. do not have adequate sidewalks. Fifty-five percent have no bike lanes or bike paths, which is partially due to poor funding.[908]

Cyclists and pedestrians experience 13 percent of annual vehicular related deaths, but a mere 1.5 percent of federal funding is spent on bike lanes, bike paths, and sidewalks. In contrast, 17 percent and 80 percent of funding is designated for public transportation and roads/highways, respectively.[909] The overwhelming majority of Americans support increased funding for sidewalks, bike lanes, and bike paths.

As for distracted cell phone drivers who cause vehicular accidents, there must be serious consequences beyond an increase in their insurance premiums. Presently, in the state of Mississippi a felony is applicable only if the driver flees the accident scene, is under the influence of alcohol, or intentionally uses his vehicle to cause injury or death.

Neither drunk drivers nor cell phone drivers intend to cause harm or death, but they both do. The drunk driver faces severe consequences for his negligence, but the cell phone driver receives a mere slap on the hand. Unless cell phone drivers face comparable criminal consequences, they will continue to be a public safety threat to everyone on the road, including drivers, cyclists, and pedestrians.

Chapter 11

The Fountain of Youth

Beyond protecting bones, regular physical activity provides other health benefits associated with aging. Overall, people who are physically active are less likely to develop and die of preventable diseases like type 2 diabetes mellitus, stroke, various forms of cancer and heart disease. They can normalize their blood pressure, glucose, cholesterol and triglycerides levels, develop a smaller waist line, lose weight, and significantly improve the health of their hearts by making it stronger.

Regular weight bearing exercises will suffice, according to various research findings. The Women's Health Initiative Observational study demonstrated that Black and White postmenopausal women of any bodyweight and age can substantially reduce their risk of developing cardiovascular disease by walking or vigorously exercising. Women in the study who walked or exercised for 30 minutes five days a week were successful at reducing their risk by 30 percent. Those who engaged in both activities experienced a reduced risk of 37 percent.(910)

Another large and long study, the Nurses' Health Study, produced comparable results. Women who engaged in either three hours of brisk walking per week or 1.5 hours of vigorous exercise per week experienced a 30 percent to 40 percent lower rate of myocardial infarction (heart attack) than sedentary women.(911)

Mental Health

Regular physical activity improves mental health and cognitive function as we age. It helps counteract the harmful effects of stress by boosting levels of serotonin and dopamine.

Exercise, mainly brisk workouts, can improve mood and treat depression. Researchers at the University of Texas Southwestern Medical Center reported that men, regardless of family history of mental illness, and women without a family history, experienced lower rates of depression when they participated in higher levels of exercise.(912)

The more a person is physically active the lower the risk of developing cognitive dysfunction. In a study that involved elderly men and women, 90 percent of the group who participated in modest light physical activity maintained their cognitive function, but those who remained sedentary did not.(913) In another study, the University of California reported that elderly women who performed higher levels of walking were less likely to experience cognitive decline.(914)

The Real Thing

"Many people falsely believe that the benefits of exercise will be found in a pill. We have clearly shown that there is no substitute for the real thing of exercise when it comes to protection from aging," stated Professor Mark Tarnopolsky, principal investigator of an exciting exercise and aging study at McMaster University in Ontario, Canada.(915)

Dr. Tarnopolsky and his colleagues have demonstrated that endurance exercise can prevent premature aging in nearly every tissue and organ system in the body and extend the lifespan. The study involved mice with genetically engineered dysfunctional mitochondria (mtDNA).

Mitochondria are "structures within cells that convert the energy from food into a form that cells can use."(916) Mitchondrial DNA helps regulate the self-destruction of cells and is necessary for the production of substances like cholesterol and hemoglobin. There are a number of conditions caused by changes in the structure of Mitochondrial DNA, including cancer, diabetes, and neuropathy. As we age, mtDNA becomes less effective and malfunctions. Consequently, our bodies begin to show the negative effects of aging, but endurance exercise can slow the adverse effects.

In the animal study, the mice were placed in two groups: one that remained sedentary and another that regularly exercised. The exercise group was engaged in five months of endurance exercise. The results were astounding. The group of mice that was sedentary aged prematurely (enlarged hearts, spindly muscles and shrunken brains) and died before reaching 1 year of age. In contrast, the physically active group, which ran 45 minutes three times a week, remained youthful at eight months and was alive at 1 year of age. Every tissue and bodily system of the exercise group had been positively impacted.[(917)]

By now, it should be clear that physical activity is a crucial component in preventing and reversing chronic diseases, protecting and restoring bones, and delaying the adverse effects associated with aging. And, it pays much higher and longer dividends than a pill.

PART IV

Living Proof

The previous chapters provided a considerable amount of scientific evidence to support the case for healthy lifestyle changes in preventing and reversing chronic diseases. However, no amount of studies is more convincing than the experiences of real people who have restored or maintained their good health by putting the evidence to practice.

This chapter presents lifestyle change experiences of a diverse group of Mississippians. They are low, middle, and upper income, uninsured and insured. The complexity of their health conditions ranged from hypertension to heart disease. There is one shared theme in their experiences. They took ownership of their health through making the necessary behavioral changes to improve their health and overall quality of life.

Chapter 12

We are the Cure

A Shot in the Dark

Susan Stonecypher is a 38 year old White female. She has traditionally eaten a very healthy mostly organic diet and has never smoked tobacco or drank alcohol. So, she was shocked to be diagnosed with multiple sclerosis (MS) at the age 27.

"I woke up one day with dim vision in my right eye," Susan said. Her optometrist prescribed eye drops, but the condition became progressively worse: fuzzy, dimmer and grayer. She returned to her physician who checked her eye and found a lesion on the optic nerve. "Your age and sex is a strong indicator of MS," she recalls him saying. The legion was later confirmed by a neuro-opthalmologist at the University of Mississippi Medical Center.

For further examination, Susan had a MRI performed at the Cleveland Clinic's Mellen Center for Multiple Sclerosis Treatment and Research in Ohio. The MRI found lesions on her brain, which confirmed that she had developed MS. She also tested positive for the Epstein Barr virus, which is a risk factor for developing MS. The physician quickly recommended that she start treatment.

"You can start preventative treatment to possibly slow the disease and prevent disability down the road," the physician explained. He was referring to Interferon beta-1a intramuscular injection, which is the standard treatment for controlling MS symptoms and slowing the development of disability, but it is no cure. The treatment causes numerous adverse effects such as: peripheral neuropathy, depression, suicidal thoughts, hallucinating, seizures, trouble breathing when lying flat in bed, stomach pain, and eye problems.(918) "All the treatments were intramuscular injections. They were all questionable. It was a shot in the dark," Susan said.

Displeased with the therapy recommendations, she decided to seek answers at the Mayo Clinic in Florida where the diagnosis was reconfirmed and the same treatment was recommended. "I was told that if I didn't take the drugs, my 5 year outlook would be a grim picture," she said. Rather than succumb to conventional wisdom, she followed her own.

She returned to Mississippi where she was referred to Dr. Ruth Fredericks, a neurologist, who she describes as a phenomenal support. Dr. Fredericks monitors her condition, and she makes suggestions. More importantly, she respects her decision not to use pharmaceutical therapies. Susan chose to take a natural and holistic approach that would involve a lifestyle change.

With the support of her husband, her first lifestyle change was resigning from her stressful job and becoming a stay-at-home mother. Additionally, her family progressed from a vegetarian diet to a vegan one. "Prior to the dietary change, I would feel a lot of fatigue and pain. I believe that the vegan diet, which is anti-inflammatory, is great for me and my doctor agrees," Susan said.

Her diet includes significantly more raw foods and no grains. Even though it's not a cure for MS, it has provided greater health benefits, according to Susan:

> I have more energy, mental clarity, restful sleep and a better digestive system. My skin is clearer, less puffy. My husband lost 10 pounds, and no one ever gets sick. It's the forever thing for us.

In addition to improving her diet, Susan uses other natural therapies to address symptoms caused by MS. For instance, she has used acupuncture for pain relief, chiropractic therapy to address fatigue, and massage therapy for relaxation. She has invested in an infrared sauna for cellular level detoxification and found it to be very peaceful and relaxing.

Susan has defied the grim forecast of his physicians. Not only is she successfully managing the disease, she has significantly improved her overall health and that of her family, which now includes another healthy son.

A Walking Medicine Cabinet

Tarah Mannery is a 38 year old Black female. She has a history of upper respiratory problems.

At 26 years of age, she began seeing a pulmonologist, a lung specialist. He prescribed antibiotics, steroids, and anti-inflammatory drugs, but the therapy was not successful, Tara explained:

> It seemed that my symptoms were not improving. At some point during that time, he tested me for rheumatoid disorders, and the lab work revealed that I had Sjogren's syndrome, disorder of the immune system that often accompanies lupus and rheumatoid arthritis. I began seeing a rheumatologist due to chronic fatigue, severe joint pain and recurring upper respiratory infections and parasthesia. He confirmed that I had Sjogren's syndrome, so he added more drug medications to my therapy. At this time I was taking up to 6 drugs daily.

She tried Plaquenil, but blindness is an adverse side-effect of the drug. So, Tarah had to get her eyes checked every 6 weeks as she was informed that her vision was diminishing.

> I feared that I would lose my eyesight eventually. I got fed up with the rheumatologist because my health was not improving. I experienced another lung infection that did not clear up and the rheumatologist sent me back to the pulmonologist who later learned that I had pneumonia, which was very bad at that point. Consequently, I had to take more steroids.

Her quality of life suffered immensely. She had become lethargic, weak, depressed, drug-induced over weight and embarrassed because of the plethora of medications she was required to take. She could barely perform her job; her supervisor had to make provisions for her at work. Even though she suffered while performing her job, she would not take sick leave because she could not afford to.

Shortly afterwards, Tarah developed with lupus-like symptoms. Over the course of 2 years, she experimented with a number of drugs to manage her symptoms. During this time, she was still experiencing upper respiratory infections caused by the immune suppressing drugs she was taking.

Enough is Enough

> One day, I was sitting home, and I looked in my book bag full of medications. I said to myself this is not the way I want to live. I knew there had to be better way towards healing. I called my friends in search of natural alternatives. It led me to a physician who practiced integrative medicine.

Her previous diet was composed of fried foods and various types of processed foods and soft drinks. She was devastated to learn of the dietary changes she would have to make. "I remember sitting in the office and putting down my head. I was like, Lord, not my ice cream." Her physician placed Tarah on a diet that excluded dairy, salt, sugar, friend foods and emphasized whole wheat, fresh vegetables, limited fruit, chicken and fish, strictly water and raw vegetable juice over a 4 week period.

Tarah followed the diet for a period of 4 weeks. After the first week, she began having withdrawal symptoms (headaches, fatigue, acne, bad sugar cravings). The second week she began feeling better, but the cravings remained. By the 3rd week, her energy level had significantly increased. Her sinus problems and skin had cleared up and the sugar cravings were history. At the end of the 4 week period, her thoughts were clearer and her energy level was very high. Nevertheless, she continued to experience joint pain and swelling.

She returned for a follow-up visit at the end of 4 weeks. Her lab work revealed that some deficiencies remained. Dr. White recommended Pregnenolone, a naturally occurring hormone. It did stop the joint pain and swelling, and it sharpened her mental clarity, but it caused acne. So, she discontinued using it.

On Her Own

Tarah began to independently investigate and try natural remedies such as garlic, fish oil, primrose oil, and Grapeseed extract. She abruptly stopped taking all her medications and became very ill. She asked the pulmonologist about reducing her medication dosage, but he advised against it. He had expected her to take the medications for life, but he did not know his patient very well as Tarah took matters into her own hands and began reducing the dosage:

> After reducing the dosage, I noticed an improvement in my joint pain. I had fewer episodes of sinus infections that I was able to clear up without antibiotics. I ate a combination of chopped raw garlic, apples, and honey. I also used sinus irrigation that helped to flush my sinuses, decrease inflammation in my nasal lining and stop a lot of the drainage, which is what caused the bronchitis that usually followed the sinus infections. I noticed that each time I would develop a sinus infection or some other upper respiratory infection I was able to clear it up without drug medications. Once I got a urinary tract infection and I used cranberry concentrate and garlic to successfully treat it, but I was still experiencing low back pain from the infection. So, I continued with my remedy, and by day 4 the back pain was alleviated.

In 2008, Tarah stopped taking her drug medications; she managed her condition with natural therapies. She felt that a physician was no longer needed until she began experiencing a shortness of breath. Her pulmonologist recommended that she resume taking steroids and Plaquenil because she was at risk of experiencing multisystem failure. This meant her lungs would shut down and eventually other organs would also. Tara was angry because she thought everything had been going so well. "Give me 2 weeks, and if I can't correct it by then I will reconsider taking the meds," she pleaded with her physician.

She saw a new rheumatologist, who informed her that Sjogren's syndrome was still in her blood, but there were not enough symptoms to be classified as having lupus. She recommended that Tarah not resume taking the medications because she was doing well.

During a regular exercise regimen, she began experiencing shortness of breath. Her physician recommended a CAT scan that showed she had a blood clot in her right lung. She reluctantly decided to take a blood thinner medication that eradicated the clot within 3 months. Her physician agreed that she could continue taking her natural cocktail. She had a follow-up CAT scan at the end of 3 months. It showed that the blood clot was not merely gone, but her physician was shocked that her lungs had not been damaged, and she had survived the ordeal. Tarah believes that garlic, a purported natural blood thinner, protected her lungs from further damage.

Presently, Tarah's natural cocktail includes flax, garlic, fish oil, primrose oil, Grapeseed extract, vitamin C, and a product called *Stress Advantage*. Her diet consists of regular juicing of fresh vegetables, and it has remained free of milk, ice cream, sugar, aspartame, and soft drinks. She limits beef and pork to 1-2 times per month.

She no longer sees a physician except for annual physical examinations. Tarah strongly advises everyone to "take responsibility for your health, listen to your doctor but always research his advice because doctors don't always know what's best," she concluded.

The Company We Keep

Rhonda Burton is a 54 year old White female. As a child she regularly ate healthy meals that primarily included vegetables, and she was very physically active:

> I played every sport that I could be involved in while in high school. We got kicked outdoors and were forced to play outside all day until the sun came down. I think that has a lot to do with how healthy most of us were. I was breastfed and received a lot of nourishing foods. I never had any childhood diseases. Unlike today's children, my sister and I received a few vaccinations.

According to Rhonda, her health problems began while she was a supervisor at a national delivery company and simultaneously attending college. "I began experiencing a jabbing pain in the right side of my stomach, which was being caused by a duodenal ulcer (H. pyloric)."

The physician prescribed Prilosec and Nexium that seemed to eradicate the ulcer, but the drugs caused severe bloating and sluggishness immediately after she ate:

> I took the drugs for about 1 year on and off. Then I stopped and I began juicing carrots, celery, apples and sometimes beets. I juiced everyday for several months. My stomach returned to a normal state of health and my energy increased.

Although she successfully used vegetables to correct the condition, she soon learned that other foods and beverages were culprits:

> If I drink alcohol (a beer or glass of wine) or eat processed foods for several consistent days, I will experience stom-

> ach pain, a sluggish feeling, painful joints and inflammation. Let's just say that now I am much more aware of what I can and cannot eat and how my health is affected by it. Primarily, I eat fresh natural whole foods (fruits, vegetables, grains, reverse osmosis water, organic chicken or beef and rarely turkey).

Rhonda's advice to others who are interested in being healthy is to regularly exercise, eat healthy, stop using tobacco, and drink alcohol in moderation. Also, she strongly believes that in order to live a healthy lifestyle we must surround ourselves with people who share our lifestyle:

> I feel that that you are or will become the person with whom you spend a lot of time socializing. For instance, if you hang out with people who drink alcohol and eat bad food, eventually you will fall into that trap. This is why it's so important for those of us who want to maintain our health to hang around like-minded people. Rather they are male or female, Black or White, all of my friends are striving to live a healthy life, and that makes it much easier for me to stay on this path.

Feeling like Superman

Johnny Minninger is a 55 year old White male. When Johnny was 10 years of age, he began experiencing very bad sinus problems. He believes his earlier life as a hay farmer exposed him to toxic chemicals that likely caused the problem or at least aggravated it:

> We didn't know about the dangers of chemicals and never wore a mask. I had recurring sinus infections for which I used many antibiotics. It would temporarily give me relief but did not cure the problem. There was scar tissue and polyps that blocked my sinus drainage.

During his 20s, his condition led to surgery. "The surgeon told me there was no other alternative to surgery," he said. After surgery, his physician administered shots that made him extremely sick. The surgery and shots were the catalyst for his healthy lifestyle change:

> I began wearing a mask in both professions (hay farmer and firefighter) or I stayed out of toxic atmospheres. I began researching natural health products to treat myself. Local bee pollen was the first thing I took, and I started on a good regimen of vitamins and minerals. Some seem to have benefits and others did not. Next, I began jogging 3 miles per week, weight training 3 times a week, and I began to pay more attention to my hydration. I moved from drinking a couple glasses of water per day to 2-3 quarts. I also began filtering the water on my refrigerator.

In addition to taking supplements and exercising, Johnny drastically changed his diet. He had been reared on a diet high in fried foods, meats, and potatoes and some vegetables:

> I developed a garden and began growing my own fruits and vegetables (tomatoes, cucumbers, watermelon, cantaloupe, onion, peppers, green beans, peas, corn, blue berries, and Blackberries) I used minimal pesticides. I began eating more fresh fruits and vegetables and moved away from white products (bleached flour, sugar, high fructose corn syrup). I ate minimal white rice, potatoes, bread, and dairy. I switched from dairy milk to almond milk because I learned that no human needs cow's milk particularly when they reach the age of 3. It's better to get your calcium from other sources such as green leafy vegetables. By the age of 30, I had eliminated soft drinks because of the high fructose corn syrup and high empty calories. When I quit drinking soft drinks I lost 20 pounds without changing anything else.

Thanks to his new lifestyle, Johnny continued to thrive without health issues until he reached his 40's. He began having some of the typical aging problems such as joint and back pain, sleeping problems, and urinary problems:

> I responded by taking glucosamine and MSM [dietary supplements] for my joints, saw palmetto, and pygeum for my prostate. Initially, there appeared to be some relief but the symptoms were never alleviated rather they progressed as I aged. When I turned 52, I was introduced to an anti-aging supplement called Protandim. Between 2 and 6 months of taking the supplement, I began sleeping like I did when I was a child and dreaming often. My prostate symptoms have been totally eradicated. Arthritic type pain in my left hip and knee is gone, and so is the tendonitis in my forearm. My weight lifting abilities have

> increased by about 50 percent. Stamina and recovery have gone through the roof. I have been able to keep up with and outpace my younger fire fighter colleagues. Taking Protandim improved my well being and overall quality of life so much that I became distributor. I also take vitamin D3, fish oil and a B complex, but I take absolutely no pharmaceutical prescription, or over-the-counter.

Johnny's healthy lifestyle has paid off for his employer as well. He has been a firefighter for about 24 years. According to him, he has accrued over 2500 hours of unused sick leave because he has never been sick. In contrast, he says the majority of his co-workers constantly utilize their sick leave because they are continuously sick. "I have never felt better in my life. I bet this is what Superman fills like."

Paramount Importance

Andrew Thomas is a 30 year old White male. Andrew has struggled with obesity most of his young life. When he graduated from high school, he weighed 360 pounds. "Everyone in my family was obese. We were all very ashamed of our bodies, but we were also addicted to the pleasure of food and television. Our lifestyle was quite sedentary," he shared.

When Andrew became a junior in college, he decided that he would take control of his weight. "I wanted to have sex, a normal life and feel confident around women. Also, I no longer wanted to be afraid of my physical inadequacies so I could play baseball with my friends," he said. Andrew took a break from college, moved out of his parents' home and got a full time job:

> Finally, I got to decide what was in my fridge. First, I focused on moving away from choosing food based upon pleasure rather health. So, I bought lots of fresh vegetables and fruits and protein powder. Next, I joined a gym and began working out regularly. I lost 130 pounds.

Even though Andrew has additional weight to lose, he is well on his way as he has created the type of healthy lifestyle to support his goal. "I am confident for the first time in my life. Now, I can take off my shirt on the beach without feeling insecure. I have performed in a play and joined an informal basketball team," he elaborated.

Along the journey, Andrew found the love of his life, Amy Breckenridge, with whom he shares his healthy lifestyle. "I feel so gratified and worthy of this relationship." Andrew continued. Amy has been great for his ego and his health. She, who is a picture of wholesome living, was living a healthy lifestyle before meeting Andrew.

Since their relationship, Andrew has lost an additional 10 pounds. Their diet is primarily plant based, organic, and locally grown. They catch and eat local fish, and Andrew has introduced Amy to eating wild game that he hunts:

> She has taught me that what I put in my body is of paramount importance. She is also very careful with the type of foods she brings home for us to eat. Our plates are small, half the size of the plates I grew up with. Now, I eat 5 small meals per day and brown bag my lunch.

Andrew has made a life time commitment to living healthy, but he admits that it is hard because he remains addicted to food:

> If I have an emotional confrontation, my first reaction is to eat something, and it's difficult to remind myself that it's a bad idea, but when I do I am successful. It has taken me a long time to understand that loving and taking care of me is my number 1 responsibility and challenge, but I believe I can stay on this path, my health, and quality of life depends on it.

Into Our Hands

Tawanna Chapman is a 34 year old Black woman. Although she has not experienced any chronic diseases, she has learned that prenatal health and infant feeding choices can substantially influence a child's health.

Becoming a young wife and mother were major motivating factors for her to adopt a healthy lifestyle. She married when she was 19 years old, and she had her first child at 20. Her family did not have private medical insurance; therefore, she was at the mercy of the public medical system.

To make matters worse, she did not know how to cook or understand the importance of eating healthy, specifically while pregnant. "I am 5'5," and during my first pregnancy I weighed 225 pounds. I was eating 2 hamburgers a day, but my physician never counseled me about eating healthy," she said.

Her physician failed to encourage and support her decision to breast-feed her son:

> I nursed my first son for only 4 months because I had problems with him latching on. I simply did not have a support system. The White lactation specialist who was assigned to help me would not come to my home, which is a Black neighborhood in Jackson, MS.

Consequently, she was forced to feed dairy based formula to her son. Within 2 months of consuming dairy formula, he began experiencing chronic ear infections:

> We were constantly going to the doctor for antibiotics. I was warned that if the infections continued, he would need tubes by age 2. So, I switched to soy formula and he had no more infections. I later learned that dairy is the number 1 allergen that causes ear infections in children.

After her first pregnancy, she made more dietary and lifestyle changes:

> I adopted a macrobiotic diet which consisted of lots of vegetables and fruits and no added sugar or junk food. I also learned to cook simple but healthy meals. If we can't make it, you won't find it in my house.

Although she became a vegetarian, her family eats turkey, chicken and sometimes lamb and fish. In addition to eating healthy, she began walking on a treadmill 1 hour every day. "We began to take our health into our hands. I was no longer willing to be at the mercy of the medical care system," she said.

Her decision to take control of her health made a huge difference in her second birthing experience at age 21:

> This time I had a healthy mind and body and a greater appreciation for the life I was carrying; I was excited. I gained merely 10-15 pounds during my second pregnancy. I continued to regularly exercise, and my husband and I took Lamaze classes.

When Tawanna became pregnant the second time, she was determined to have a healthier and more natural birthing experience. So, she replaced her physician with a midwife and the hospital with her home:

> My midwife helped me to address food cravings and the at-home visits included massage therapy, reflexology and regular prenatal care. I had a totally natural birth and breastfed my son for two and a half years.

Today, Tawanna is a veteran of healthy cooking and the primary provider of her family's health. Her family sees the doctor once a year for physical exams. When the rare health issue arises, it tends to be mild and short in duration:

> I know I will live the rest of my life being conscious of my health. Even though nothing is guaranteed, I believe that healthy living will at a minimum greatly improve my chances of not getting sick and dying early.

Doctor Mom

Linda Jackson is a 54 year old Black female. She is a wonderful example of how healthy living can build and maintain good health and slow aging.

She has never had a chronic disease, and she has rarely used drug medications. She uses healthy behavior to prevent illnesses and natural remedies to treat rare conditions.

> I am doctor mom in my home. Health for me and my family is a way of life. By that I mean eating healthy, exercising, and handling stress through talking and laughing. We treat minor illnesses such as colds with homeopathic and herbal medicines, and we see a doctor once a year for a physical exam. I feel strongly that our lifestyle, especially our vegetarian diet, protects our health from obesity and diseases like type 2 diabetes, which are running rampant in Mississippi.

Linda became a vegetarian 20 years ago because she saw the negative effects of unhealthy eating in her community. Her diet primarily consists of fish, beans, grains, nuts, and soy. Although she has removed meat from her diet, she has not been able to overcome her love for sweets:

> My struggle is sugar (desserts), but I have reduced the portion size. I drink huge amounts of water and occasionally sweet tea and 100 fruit juice. I also control what I eat by cooking meals at home. My goal is to reach 100 years of age. I know there are no guarantees, but it's my responsibility and choice to do everything I can to stay healthy as long as I possibly can. I believe a healthy lifestyle will help me to reach my goal.

Gary Griffin

Gary Griffin is a 54 year old Black man. When he turned 51 his physician presented him with a diagnosis of pre-diabetes, and congestive heart failure. His heart was functioning at 67 percent capacity. Several expensive medications were prescribed as well as a very much needed lifestyle change.

The news was disappointing but not a complete surprise as Gary had smoked *Kool* and *Newport* menthol cigarettes for nearly 40 years. In addition to being addicted to cigarettes, he regularly consumed fast foods and fried foods. According to him, his life was typically stressful because of his commitment to everyone except himself. Yet, Gary was driven by a strong desire to stick around to enjoy his family, which propelled him to make the immediate lifestyle changes to save his life.

For instance, tobacco cessation experts taught him new behaviors to quit smoking.

- chewing nicorette gum,
- maintaining a toothpick in his mouth,
- refraining from drinking coffee, which was previously accompanied with a cigarette,
- placing the cigarette packages in the trunk of his vehicle to prevent easy access while driving.

In addition to being a smoker, Gary was over-weight, especially around his abdominal section. He instantly replaced fast foods with home cooked meals that included significantly more vegetables, fruits, fish, and poultry. And, he reduced his caloric intake to 1200 per day.

He swapped unhealthy snacks with healthy alternatives at home and in the workplace. The three soft drinks he drank daily were replaced with 1 gallon of water. Now, he drinks soft drinks on rare occasions. Gary supplements his new diet with daily tablespoon of fish oil and an aspirin.

Along with dietary changes, he increased his level of physical activity to 45 minutes per day. He began taking the stairs, riding a bike, walking, and lifting weights.

Over a 3-month period, Gary was able to stop taking his medications, and within 9 months he lost 18 pounds. Today, his heart is functioning at 72 percent capacity. He realizes that he has to continue to live healthy to fully restore his heart:

> At the rate I was going, I would have had a stroke, heart attack, or died. After making the necessary changes, which are much more affordable than those prescribed meds, I have increased clarity and energy, but I must continue on this path so that my heart will function at 100 percent. Overall I simply feel much better. I am also more productive at home and work. I don't allow stress to bother me as much as I used to because I no longer try to control the outcomes of actions taken by my family or me.

Chapter 13

Putting it to the Test

One of the most powerful and captivating questions ever uttered by a movie character was that of Jim Malone in the *Untouchables.* As he lay dying on the floor barely able to speak, Malone passionately grabbed Eliot Ness by the collar and handed him a crucial piece of evidence to defeat his nemesis, Al Capone. He asked Ness, "What are you prepared to do? What are you prepared to do?"

At some point in our lives, we are presented with crucial information that can change the outcome of a critical situation. That information challenges us to take action. In this instance, you are being asked to evaluate your lifestyle and make the necessary changes to prevent and reverse chronic diseases. The link between unhealthy behavior and disease has been established, and the solutions are presented through numerous studies in which healthy lifestyle changes proved to be equally or more effective than drugs and surgeries.

You have learned about the vital role that risk factors like abdominal obesity, sweetened beverages, processed foods, excessive alcohol, and tobacco play in developing and reversing chronic diseases. Finally, you have read the stories of a diverse group of people who have restored their health through healthy lifestyle changes. Isn't it time you put healthy living to the test? You can begin by creating a lifestyle change plan.

Lifestyle Change Plan

In getting started, you should consider including your family, friends, neighbors, or co-workers as they likely share similar risk factors. Their participation and support can improve your chance of being successful.

Take the following steps to develop your personal lifestyle change plan:

1. Complete the Metabolic Syndrome Health Risk Assessment (MSHRA) located at the end of this chapter. If you have 3 or more of the risk factors, you are at significant risk of developing type 2 diabetes and cardiovascular disease.

2. If you have not had a physical examination in the last 12 months, get one. If you don't have medical insurance or adequate funds, consider going to a federally funded community clinic and enrolling in the *Health Insurance Market Place.*

3. Tell your health care provider that you have decided to implement a healthy lifestyle change plan. This is an opportunity to build a partnership with your provider. Ask for suggestions. If your health care provider shuns this approach, find one who will support you. A good health care provider should not encourage you to remain on chronic disease medication for an indefinite period of time rather he should encourage and help you to make the necessary changes that will eventually take you off drug medications.

4. Use the results of your physical exam and MSHRA to determine your personal health goal(s). For example, your personal health goal may be to lower your blood pressure, LDL level, bodyweight, or to increase your HDL level. Keep in mind that when you make healthy lifestyle changes to prevent or correct one condition, other conditions are often corrected as well. For instance, the lifestyle changes you make to lose body weight will likely lower your LDL, glucose, and blood pressure levels.

5. Observe your typical day and figure out how you can turn obstacles into opportunities for change. For instance, your work schedule may pose a problem for exercising or your worksite does not have a wellness program. Your goal is to find a way to overcome barriers. That may require getting up 30 minutes earlier, going to bed 30 minutes later or using your lunch to exercise. It may require joining a group fitness class or better yet, approaching your employer about allowing you and your co-workers to develop a wellness program within the worksite. Remember, barriers are opportunities for change.

6. If you are a smoker seek out smoking cessation programs at your place of employment or nonprofit community organizations. Again, if your employer does not offer tobacco cessation counseling, this is an opportunity to suggest that a worksite wellness program be created. Meanwhile, you can begin setting limitations on your smoking. For instance, getting rid of ashtrays is a good start.

7. Once you have completed the previous steps, complete the *Personal Lifestyle Change Plan* form. The purpose of this form is to help you organize your plan.

Your New Diet

Your new diet should be nutritionally rich and designed to help you maintain your overall good health. There is no point in adopting a diet to target a particular chronic disease because a healthy diet that can prevent hypertension also can prevent type 2 diabetes and coronary heart disease. That is a diet high in fresh foods but low in processed foods. Remember, processed foods and beverages are high in fructose corn syrup, sugar, and sodium and low in vitamins and minerals. An excellent nutritional source is the World's Healthiest Foods, atwww.whfoods.com. It is an extensive database of scientifically proven nutritional information, including healthy recipes.[(886)]

Eating fresh foods is the best way to treat nutritional deficiencies. The human body needs 13 vitamins: vitamins A, C, D, E, K, and B vitamins (thiamine, riboflavin, niacin, pantothenic acid, biotin, vitamin B-6, vitamin B-12 and folate). Macrominerals and trace minerals are important as well. Macrominerals, which your body needs in relatively large amounts, include: calcium, magnesium, sodium, phosphorus, potassium, sulfur, and chloride. Iron, copper, iodine, manganese, zinc, cobalt, selenium, and fluoride are trace minerals that are needed in small amounts.

A comprehensive micro-nutritional test will identify vitamin, mineral, and antioxidant deficiencies. Ask your medical provider or check out Spectra Cell Labs. It offers a comprehensive nutrition assessment that is covered by insurance with a doctor's order or you can order online at www.spectracell.com.

Read food labels when shopping for processed foods. Remember, ingredients are listed in descending order by weight. So, be wary of front labels that may make false and misleading claims about the nutritional quality of the product. The only way you can be sure you are buying a whole food product is by reading the ingredient label.

For example, the following are various names of added sugar found on ingredient lists:

> Agave nectar, brown sugar, cane crystals, cane sugar, corn sweetener, corn syrup, crystalline fructose, dextrose, evaporated cane juice, fructose, fruit juice concentrates, glucose, high-fructose corn syrup, honey, invert sugar, lactose, maltose, malt syrup, molasses, raw sugar, sucrose, sugar, and syrup.

As a guide, I strongly recommend that you use Harvard University's *Healthy Eating Plate,* not the USDA *MyPlate,* which appears to be primarily aligned with federally subsidized foods. For example, the *Healthy Eating Plate* specifies healthy whole grains and limits refined grains, but

MyPlate generalizes grains. *MyPlate* does not distinguish between healthy protein choices, e.g. salmon and red meat or processed meats. In contrast, the *Healthy Eating Plate* specifies fish, poultry, beans or nuts, and it discourages frequently eating red meat and all processed meats. *MyPlate* recommends dairy with every meal, and it makes no mention of sugary beverages. The *Healthy Eating Plate* recommends water, restricting dairy consumption, avoiding sugary beverages and limiting 100 percent fruit juice. Healthy oils are excluded on *MyPlate.*

Finally, the *Healthy Eating Plate* recommends physical activity, but *MyPlate* does not. Although neither guide recommends it, you should eat organic foods when possible.

Eating Organic Foods

A number of studies have identified organically grown foods as having higher levels of antioxidants.[920-924]

Antioxidants are substances that counteract the negative effects of free radicals, which cause damage at the cellular level and increase the risk of developing chronic and degenerative diseases such as diabetes, cardiovascular disease and cancer. Antioxidants tend to be plentiful in plant based foods, especially fruits, vegetables, and nuts, but some foods have higher levels than others. Moreover, these antioxidant rich foods may need to be regularly consumed and in large amounts to produce beneficial effects.

For example, a study conducted by researchers at the United States Department of Agriculture's Arkansas Children's Nutrition Center found that eating at least a half-cup to more than one cup of blueberries, mixed grapes, and especially kiwi produced an increase in blood plasma antioxidant capacity. Consuming one and one-third cup of the fruits produced the highest level of antioxidant volume.[925]

In addition to providing higher antioxidant levels, organically grown foods have been shown to be safer in that these foods have significantly fewer pesticide residues.[926] Children who primarily consume organic foods have a significantly lower exposure to organophosphorus pesticide.[927] Organophosphorus compounds are highly toxic and inhibit the effectiveness of natural killer (NK) cells.

The President's Cancer Panel's advises Americans to reduce their risk of developing cancer by eating organic foods and free range meat[928]:

> Exposure to pesticides can be decreased by choosing, to the extent possible, food grown without pesticides or chemical fertilizers and washing conventionally grown produce to remove residues. Similarly, exposure to antibiotics, growth hormones, and toxic run-off from livestock feed lots can be minimized by eating free-range meat raised without these medications if it is available. Avoiding or minimizing consumption of processed, charred, and well-done meats will reduce exposure to carcinogenic heterocyclic amines and polyaromatic hydrocarbons.

The fact that organic food sales have reached $27 billion[929] strongly suggests a significant number of Americans are concerned about environmental toxins in their foods. Consumption of organic fresh meat, poultry, and seafood has nearly tripled in the U.S.

The following are FDA rules regarding organic foods:[930-931]:

1. Antibiotics are banned in animals that are intended for human food consumption. Organic feed and water must be free of antibiotics and hormones. If an animal becomes sick and receives antibiotics, it cannot be sold as organic. This includes milk from dairy cows treated with antibiotics.

2. Recombinant bovine somatotropin (rBST), a synthetic hormone used in dairy cows, is banned in organic dairy cows.

3. Arsenic and sodium nitrate are not allowed in organic livestock, particularly, chickens.

4. Food additives and processing aids (MSG, colorings, artificial sweeteners, preservatives, and flavorings) are banned or severely restricted in organic foods.

5. Synthetic pesticides (insecticides, fungicides and herbicides) are prohibited in organic crops and animals, all stages of organic food production, handling and processing.

6. Genetically Modified Organisms (GMOs) are not permitted in organic foods.

7. Food irradiation is not allowed in organic products.

Do not confuse labels claiming to be ***natural*** with ***organic***. The USDA does not regulate or guarantee labels claiming to be natural. These foods could have a few natural ingredients among a long list of additives and/or genetically modified foods (GMOs). Look for the ***USDA 100 percent Organic*** seal to be sure you're getting the real thing. It applies to raw, fresh, and processed organic foods that are made of organic agricultural ingredients.

Also, remember, all labels claiming to be organic are not totally organic. For instance, excluding water and salt, products labeled "***100 percent organic***" must exclusively contain organically produced ingredients and processing aids. In contrast, those merely labeled "***organic***" are required to contain a minimum of 95 percent organic ingredients, excluding salt and water. Processed products that are made of at least 70 percent organic ingredients may be labeled "***made with organic ingredients,***" and list a maximum of 3 of the ingredients. Processed foods that contain less than 70 percent cannot use the organic label.

Physical Activity

Determine what types of physical activity you intend to incorporate in your new lifestyle. Purchase a fitness magazine such as *Oxygen* and *Men's Fitness* that are filled with simple and effective strength bearing exercises to help you lose weight and tone up.

Do not buy weight loss products that promise to help you lose weight while maintaining a sedentary lifestyle and poor diet. On the other hand, don't get overly excited and abruptly join a gym without a work out partner or coach. Also, the local college gym will likely be more affordable than privately owned gyms. You also can consider creating a gym within your home or worksite.

Be sure to incorporate weights in your workout. Lifting weights will not only tone your body and define your muscles but protect your bones by increasing bone density, which helps prevent osteoporosis, and reduce the chance of falls. Lifting improves posture, balance, and prevents muscle mass loss as we get older.

Don't forget to take a 30-minute brisk walk every day. Look for and create opportunities to walk while at work. Consider using your lunch hour or 15 minute work breaks, and get your co-workers to join you. You can lead your family and neighbors on a daily walk during the evening hours after dinner. Adopt a dog.

When possible, take the stairs, and park farther away from the entrance to your work place and other buildings. Buy bikes and helmets for you and your family and schedule regular rides in your neighborhood or bike path. Invite your neighbors to join you.

Join an outdoor club such as cycling, walking, hiking, swimming, etc. If there isn't one in your neighborhood, consider it as an opportunity to organize one. Plan regular neighborhood cycling and walking events.

As mentioned earlier, if your place of employment does not have a worksite wellness program, consider starting one with a group of coworkers. You can start small and gradually expand it. You will need the approval, support, and preferably involvement of senior management. You may need to educate management about the significant financial savings, increased productivity, and reduced absenteeism associated with a worksite wellness program. And, don't forget to include a lactation program for expecting moms. For more information on how to build a worksite wellness program, check out the CDC's Work@Health Program at http://www.cdc.gov/workathealth.

Finally, remember that living healthy is a life time commitment. You must replace the old lifestyle responsible for the existing and imminent chronic disease with one that can prevent or reverse it. As with anything else, if you remain steadfast, you will achieve amazing results over short and long term periods. The most important thing is to take control of your health and begin to make modest healthy choices. There is no better time to start than now.

We are the cure.

Metabolic Syndrome Health Risk Assessment

Metabolic Syndrome is a cluster of health conditions that increases your risk of developing coronary heart disease, stroke, and diabetes. If you have 3 or more risk factors, you are at significant risk of developing type 2 diabetes and cardiovascular disease. Please answer by placing a √.

Large waist circumference

(bulging waistline, or an "apple" belly shape)

For women, is your waist circumference 35 or greater? ❑Yes ❑No

For men, is your waist circumference 40 or greater? ❑Yes ❑No

Low level of good cholesterol (HDL)

Is your HDL less than 50 mg/dl? ❑Yes ❑No

High triglyceride level (fat in the blood)

Is your triglyceride level greater or equal to 150 mg/dl? ❑Yes ❑No

High Fasting Plasma Glucose (blood sugar)

Is your fasting glucose level 100 mg/dL or greater ❑Yes ❑No

High Blood Pressure

Is your blood pressure 130/85 mmHg or higher? ❑Yes ❑No

Your Total Risk Factors: ________

Next, when you are serious about making changes to improve your health, complete the *Healthy Lifestyle Change Plan.*

Lifestyle Change Plan

My personal health goal(s) is to:

The changes I will make to reach my goal(s) are:

Each day and throughout the day I will make a conscious decision to choose healthy food, drinks, and behavior that will improve and protect my health. My signature represents the beginning of my commitment to being healthy for the rest of my life.

Your Signature Date

Notes

1. Mathews TJ, MacDorman MF. Infant Mortality Statistics From the 2008 Period Linked Birth/Infant Death Data Set. National Vital Statistics Reports. Hyattsville, MD: National Center for Health Statistics. Center for Disease Control and Prevention; 2012. http://www.cdc.gov.
2. Miniño AM, Murphy SL. Death in the United States, *2010 NCHS Data Brief.* Hyattsville, MD: National Center for Health Statistics;2012. http://www.cdc.gov.
3. Top Programs in the U.S. 1995 - 2011. Washington, DC: Environmental Working Group; 2013. http://www.farm.ewg.org.
4. Top Programs in the U.S. 1995 - 2011. Washington, DC: Environmental Working Group; 2013. http://www.farm.ewg.org.
5. Dreifus C. *A Mathematical Challenge to Obesity: A conversation with Carson Chow.* New York, NY: New York Times Newspaper; 2012 May 14. http://www.nytimes.com.
6. Moneiro C. The big issue is ultra-processing. *World Nutrition.* 2010;1(6):237-269. http://www.wphna.org.
7. Monteiro C. In praise of the shared meal. *World Nutrition.*2011;2(5). http://www.wphna.org.
8. *Top Ten Facts in 2012. Mississippi Restaurant Industry At A Glance.* Washington, DC: National Restaurant Association; 2012. http://www.restaurant.org.
9. Schlosser E. *Fast Food Nation: The Dark Side of the All-American Meal.* New York: NY: Harper Collins Publishers, 2002.
10. *2005 Chain Restaurant Industry Review.* Scottsdale, AZ: Commercial Finance GE; http://www.cefcorp.com/commequip/documents/2005FranchiseIndustryReview.pdf.
11. Oches. S. The QSR 50. *Journalistic Inc.* http://www.qsrmagazine.com.
12. Harris JL, et. al. *Fast Food FACTS:* Evaluating fast food nutrition and marketing to youth. New Haven. CT: Yale University's Rudd Center for Food Policy and Obesity; 2010. http://www.rwif.org.

13. *My heart, my life.TM supporters and sponsors.* Dallas, TX: American Heart Association; 2012. http://www.heart.org.

14. *Heart Healthy Meals.* Milford, CT: Subway;2013. http:// www.subway.com.

15. American Heart Association's New Heart-Check Meal Certification Offers Consumer Confidence on Healthy Choices. Dallas, TX: American Heart Association, 2012. http://www.newsroomheart.org.

16. Lesser LI, et al. Adolescent purchasing behavior at McDonald's and Subway. *J Adolesc Health.* 2013;53(4):441-5. http://www.ncbi.nlm.nih.gov.

17. Product ingredient guide and U.S. allergy and sensitivity information. Milford, CT: Subway; June 2014. http://www.subway.com.

18. Subway® U.S. Nutrition Information. Milford, CT: Subway; March 2014. http://www.subway.com.

19. Currie J, DellaVigna S, Moretti E, Pathania V. The effect of fast food restaurants on Ooesity. 2009. http://www.emlab.berkely.edu.

20. Chou S, Grossman M, Saffer H. An economic analysis of adult obesity: Results from the behavioral risk factor surveillance system. *Journal of Health Economics.* 2004; 23(3):565-587. http://www.ncbi.nlm.nih.gov.

21. Bowman SA, Vinyard BT. Fast food consumption of U.S. adults: Impact on energy and nutrient intakes and overweight status. *J Am Coll Nutr.* 2004;23(2):163-8. http://www.ncbi.nlm.nih.gov.

22. Garcia G, Sunil TS, Hinojosa P. The fast food and obesity link: consumption patterns and severity of obesity. *Obes Surg.* 2012;22(5):810-8. http://www.ncbi.nlm.nih.gov.

23. Dunn RA, Sharkey JR, Horel S. The effect of fast-food availability on fast-food consumption and obesity among rural residents: an analysis by race/ethnicity. *Econ Hum Biol.* 2012 Jan;10(1):1-13. http://www.ncbi.nlm.nih.gov.

24. Fleischhacker SE, Evenson KR, Rodriguez DA, Ammerman AS. A systematic review of fast food access studies. *Obes Rev.* 2011 May;12(5):e460-71. http://www.ncbi.nlm.nih.gov.

25. Fraser LK, Edwards KL, Cade JE, Clarke GP. Fast food, other food choices and body mass index in teenagers in the United Kingdom (ALSPAC): a structural equation modelling approach. *Int J Obes (Lond).* 2011;35(10):1325-30. http://www.ncbi.nlm.nih.gov/pubmed/21712805.

26. Currie J, DellaVigna S, Moretti E, Pathania V. *The effect of fast food restaurants on obesity.* Jan 2009. http:// www.emlab.berkely.edu.

27. Inagami S, Cohen DA, Brown AF, Asch S. Body mass index, neighborhood fast food and restaurant concentration, and car ownership. *J Urban Health.* 2009;86(5):683–695. http://www.ncbi.nlm.nih.gov.

28. Yancey AK, Cole BL, Brown R, et al. A cross-sectional prevalence study of ethnically targeted and general audience outdoor obesity-related advertising. *Milbank Q.* 2009 ;87(1):155-84. http://www.ncbi.nlm.nih.gov/pubmed.

29. Powell LM, Chaloupka FJ, Bao Y. The availability of fast-food and full-service restaurants in the United States: associations with neighborhood characteristics. *Am J Prev Med.* 2007;33(4 Suppl):S240-5. http://www.ncbi.nlm.nih.gov.

30. Kwate, NO. Fried chicken and fresh apples: racial segregation as a fundamental cause of fast food density in black neighborhoods. *Health Place.* 2008;14(1):32-44. http://www.ncbi.nlm.nih.gov.

31. State & county quickfacts. Washington, DC: US Census Bureau. Department of Commerce; 2012. http://www.quickfacts.census.gov.

32. Hickson DA, Diez Roux AV, Smith AE, et al. Associations of fast food restaurant availability with dietary intake and weight among African Americans in the Jackson Heart Study, 2000-2004. *Am J Public Health.* 2011;101(Suppl 1):S301-9. http://www.ncbi.nlm.nih.gov.

33. Block JP, Scribner RA, DeSalvo KB. Fast food, race/ethnicity, and income: a geographic analysis. Am J Prev Med. 2004;27(3):211-7. http://www.ncbi.nlm.nih.gov.

34. Sugars & sweeteners overview. Washington DC: USDA Economic Research Service. United States of Agriculture; 2012. http://www.ers.usda.gov.

35. Putnam JJ, Allshouse JE. Food consumption, prices, and expenditures, 1970–97. Food and Consumers Economics Division, Economic Research Service, US Department of Agriculture; Washington, DC: 1999. http://www.ers.usda.gov.

36. Jacobson, MF. Liquid Candy: How soft drinks are hurting Americans' health. Washington DC: Center for the Public Interest; 2005. http://www.cspinet.org.

37. Lopes M, Prentice C. U.S. corn syrup makers slash prices to fend off cheap sugar. Chicago, IL: *Chicago Tribune Newspaper*; November 12, 2013 http://www.articles.chicagotribune.com.

38. High Fructose Corn Syrup Produce and Prices. Washington, DC: Economic Research Service. USDA; 2012. http://www.ers.usda.gov.

39. High-Fructose Corn Syrup Production and Prices. USDA. Washington, DC: Economic Research Service. USDA; 2012. http://www.ers.usda.gov.

40. High-Fructose Corn Syrup Production and Prices. Washington, DCz; Economic Research Service.USDA; 2012. http://www.ers.usda.gov.

41. Bocarsly ME, Powell ES, Avena NM, Hoebel BG. High-fructose corn syrup causes characteristics of obesity in rats: increased body weight, body fat and triglyceride levels. *Pharmacol Biochem Behav.* 2010:97(1): 101–6. http://www.ncbi.nlm.nih.gov.

42. Tou JC. The type of caloric sweetner added to water influences weight gain gain, fat mass, and reproduction in growing Sprague-Dawley rats. Exp Biol Med (Maywood).2009;234(5):651-61. http://www.ncbi.nlm.nih.gov.

43. Bray G, Nielsen S, Popkin, B. Consumption of high fructose corn syrup in beverages may play a role in the epidemic of obesity. *American Journal of Clinical Nutrition,* 2004; 79(4): 537-43. http://www.ncbi.nlm.nih.gov.

44. Smith TA, Lin BH, Lee JY. *Taxing Caloric Sweetened Beverages: Potential Effects on Beverage Consumption, Calorie Intake, and Obesity.* Washington DC: Economic Research Service/USDA; 2012. http://www.www.ers.usda.gov.

45. Ludwig DS, Peterson KE, Gortmaker SL. Relation between consumption of sugar-sweetened drinks and childhood obesity: A prospective, observational analysis. *Lancet.* 2001;357:505–508. http://www.ncbi.nlm.nih.gov.

46. Janssens JP, Shapira N, Debeuf P, et al. Effects of soft drink and table beer consumption on insulin response in normal teenagers and carbohydrate drink in youngsters. *Eur J Cancer Prev.* 1999;8:289–295. http://www.ncbi.nlm.nih.gov.

47. Malik VS, Popkin BM, Bray GA, Després JP, Willett WC, Hu FB. Sugar-sweetened beverages and risk of metabolic syndrome and type 2 diabetes: a meta-analysis. *Diabetes Care.* 2010;33(11):2477-83. http://www.ncbi.nlm.nih.gov.

48. Bhupathiraju SN, et al. Caffeinated and caffeine-free beverages and risk of type 2 diabetes. *Am J Clin Nutr.* 2013;97(1):155-66. http://www.ncbi.nlm.nih.gov.

49. Koning L, Malik VS, Rimm EB, Willett WC, Hu FB. Sugar-sweetened and artificially sweetened beverage consumption and risk of type 2 diabetes in men1. *Am J Clin Nutr.* 2011; 93(6): 1321–1327. http://www.ncbi.nlm.nih.gov.

50. Schulze MB, et al. Sugar-sweetened beverages, weight gain, and incidence of type 2 diabetes in young and middle-aged women. *JAMA.* 2004;292(8):927-34. http://www.ncbi.nlm.nih.gov.

51. Ogden CL, Kit BK, Carrol MD, Park S. *Consumption of Sugar Drinks in the United States, 2005–2008. NCHS data brief, no 71.* Hyattsville, MD: National Center for Health Statistics; 2011. http://www.cdc.gov.

52. Diabetes Statistics: Race and ethnic differences in prevalence of diagnosed diabetes. Alexandria, VA: American Diabetes Association; 2001. http://www.diabetes.org.

53. West DS, Bursac Z, Quimby D, et al. Self-reported sugar-sweetened beverage intake among college students. *Obesity (Silver Spring).* 2006;14(10):1825-31. http://www.ncbi.nlm.nih.gov.

54. Palmer JR, Boggs DA, Krishnan S, Hu FB, Singer M, Rosenberg L. Sugar-sweetened beverages and incidence of type 2 diabetes mellitus in African American women. *Arch Intern Med.* 2008;168(14):1487-92. http://www.ncbi.nlm.nih.gov.

55. High Blood Pressure Facts. Atlanta, GA: Centers for Disease Control and Prevention (CDC); 2013. http://www.cdc.gov.

56. Gao X, Qi L, Qiao N, Choi HK, Curhan G, Tucker KL, Ascherio A. Intake of added sugar and sugar-sweetened drink and serum uric acid concentration in US men and women. *Hypertension*. 2007;50(2):306-12. http://www.ncbi.nlm.nih.gov.

57. Choi JW, Ford ES, Gao X, Choi HK. Sugar-sweetened soft drinks, diet soft drinks, and serum uric acid level: the third national health and nutrition examination survey. *Arthritis Rheum. 2008;59(1):109-16.* http://www.ncbi.nlm.nih.gov.

58. Rebello T, Hodges RE, Smith JL. Short-term effects of various sugars on antinatriuresis and blood pressure changes in normotensive young men. *Am J Clin Nutr.* 1983;38(1):84-94. http://www.ncbi.nlm.nih.gov.

59. Bocarsly ME, Powell ES, Avena NM, Hoebel BG. High-fructose corn syrup causes characteristics of obesity in rats: increased body weight, body fat and triglyceride levels. *Pharmacol Biochem Behav.* 2010;97(1):101-6. http://www.ncbi.nlm.nih.gov

60. Bray GA, Nielsen SJ, Popkin BM. Consumption of high-fructose corn syrup in beverages may play a role in the epidemic of obesity. *Am J Clin Nutr. 2004;79:537–543.* http://www.ncbi.nlm.nih.gov.

61. Johnson RJ, Segal MS, Sautin Y, et al. Potential role of sugar (fructose) in the epidemic of hypertension, obesity and the metabolic syndrome, diabetes, kidney disease, and cardiovascular disease. *Am J Clin Nutr.* 2007;86(4):899-906. http://www.ncbi.nlm.nih.gov.

62. Forman JP, Choi H, Curhan GC. Uric Acid and Insulin Sensitivity and Risk of Incident Hypertension. *Arch Intern Med.* 2009; 169(2): 155–162. http://www.ncbi.nlm.nih.gov.

63. Imazu M, Yamamoto H, Toyofuku M, et al. Hyperinsulinemia for the development of hypertension: data from the Hawaii-Los Angeles-Hiroshima Study. *Hypertens Res. 2001;24(5):531-6.* http://www.ncbi.nlm.nih.gov.

64. Jossa F, Farinaro E, Panico S, et al. Serum uric acid and hypertension: the Olivetti heart study. *J Hum Hypertens.* 1994;8(9):677-81. http://www.ncbi.nlm.nih.gov.

65. Masuo K, Kawaguchi H, Mikami H, Ogihara T, Tuck ML. Serum uric acid and plasma norepinephrine concentrations predict subsequent weight gain and blood pressure elevation. *Hypertension*. 2003;42:474–80. http://www.ncbi.nlm.nih.gov.

66. Goldstein HS, Manowitz P. Relation between serum uric acid and blood pressure in adolescents. *Ann Hum Biol.* 1993;20(5):423-31. http://www.ncbi.nlm.nih.gov.

67. Ford ES, Li C, Cook S, Choi HK. Serum concentrations of uric acid and the metabolic syndrome among US children and adolescents. *Circulation.* 2007;115(19):2526-32. http://www.ncbi.nlm.nih.gov.

68. Nguyen S, Choi HK, Lustig, RH, Hsu C. Sugar sweetened beverages, serum uric acid, and blood pressure in adolescents. *J Pediatr.* 2009; 154(6): 807–813. http://www.ncbi.nlm.nih.gov.

69. Snieder H, Harshfield GA, Treiber FA. Heritability of blood pressure and hemodynamics in African- and European-American youth. *Hypertension.* 2003;41(6):1196-201. http://www.ncbi.nlm.nih.gov.

70. Savoca MR, Evans CD, Wilson ME, Harshfield GA, Ludwig DA. The association of caffeinated beverages with blood pressure in adolescents. *Arch Pediatr Adolesc Med.* 2004;158(5):473-7. http://www.ncbi.nlm.nih.gov.

71. Alper AB Jr, Chen W, Yau L, Srinivasan SR, Berenson GS, Hamm LL. Childhood uric acid predicts adult blood pressure: the Bogalusa Heart Study. *Hypertension.* 2005;45(1):34-8. http://www.ncbi.nlm.nih.gov.

72. *What Is Gout? Fast Facts: An Easy-to-Read Series of Publications for the Public.* Bethesda, MD: National Institute of Arthritis and Musculoskeletal Diseases; 2010. http://www.niams.nih.gov.

73. Choi HK, Willett W, Curhan G. Fructose-Rich Beverages and the Risk of Gout in Women. *JAMA.* 2010;304(20):2270–2278. http://www.ncbi.nlm.nih.gov.

74. Choi HK, Curhan G. Soft drinks, fructose consumption, and the risk of gout in men: prospective cohort study. *BMJ.* 2008; 336(7639): 309–312. http://www.ncbi.nlm.nih.gov.

75. Choi HK, Curhan G. Soft drinks, fructose consumption, and the risk of gout in men: prospective cohort study. *BMJ.* 2008;336(7639):309-12. http://www.ncbi.nlm.nih.gov.

76. Choi HK, Willett W, Curhan G. Fructose-rich beverages and gout in women. JAMA. 2010;304(20):2270-8. http://www.ncbi.nlm.nih.gov.

77. Fung TT, Malik V, Rexrode KM, Manson JE, Willett WC, Hu FB. Sweetened beverage consumption and risk of coronary heart disease in women. *Am J Clin Nutr.* 2009;89:1037–1042. http://www.ncbi.nlm.nih.gov.

78. de Koning L, Malik VS, Kellogg MD, Rimm EB, Willett WC, Hu FB. Sweetened Beverage Consumption, Incident Coronary Heart Disease, and Biomarkers of Risk in Men. *Circulation.* 2012;125(14):1735-41, S1.

79. Bernstein AM, Koning LD, Flint AJ, Rexrode KM, Willett WC. Soda consumption and the risk of stroke in men and women. *Am J Clin Nutr.* 2012; 95(5): 1190–1199. http://www.ncbi.nlm.nih.gov.

80. Tucker KL, Morita K, Qiao N, Hannan MT, Cupples LA, Kiel DP. Colas, but not other carbonated beverages, are associated with low bone mineral density in older women: The Framingham Osteoporosis Study. *Am J Clin Nutr.* 2006;84(4):936-42. http://www.ncbi.nlm.nih.gov.

81. Whiting SJ, Healey A, Psiuk S, et al. Relationship between carbonated and other low nutrient dense beverages and bone mineral content of adolescents. *Nutrition Research.* 200;21(8):1107-1115. http://www.ncbi.nlm.nih.gov.

82. Ma D, Jones G. Soft drink and milk consumption, physical activity, bone mass, and upper limb fractures in children: a population-based case-control study. *Calcif Tissue Int.* 2004;75(4):286-91. http://www.ncbi.nlm.nih.gov.

83. Wyshak G. Teenaged girls, carbonated beverage consumption, and bone fractures. *Arch Pediatr Adolesc Med.* 2000;154(6):610-3. http://www.ncbi.nlm.nih.gov.

84. Teenaged girls, carbonated beverage consumption, and bone fractures. *Arch Pediatr Adolesc Med. 2000;154(6):610-3.* http://www.ncbi.nlm.nih.gov.

85. Excessive Alcohol Use: A Largely Unrecognized Public Health Problem. Atlanta, GA: Centers for Disease Control and Prevention; 2011. http://www.ncbi.nlm.nih.gov.

86. Singal AK, Anand BS. Recent trends in the epidemiology of alcoholic liver disease. *Clinical Liver Disease.*2013;2(2):53-56. http://www.ncbi.nlm.nih.gov.

87. Annual Report Fiscal Year Ending June 30, 2011. Office of Alcohol Beverage Control 45 Year Comparison of Revenue Collections and Volume Sales. Jackson, MS: Mississippi Department of Revenue;2011. http://www.dor.ms.gov.

88. Sacks JJ, et al. State costs of excessive alcohol consumption, 2006. *Am J Prev Med.* 2013;45(4):474-85. http://www.ncbi.nlm.nih.gov.

89. Average for Mississippi 2006-2010 - Alcohol-Attributable Deaths Due to Excessive Alcohol Use. Atlanta, GA: National Center for Chronic Disease Prevention and Health Promotion. http://www.cdc.gov.

90. Traffic Safety Performance (Core Outcomes) Measures for Mississippi. Washington, DC: U.S. Department of Transportation; 2012. http://www-nrd.nhtsa.dot.gov.

91. Daytime and nighttime seatbelt use by fatally injured passenger vehicle occupants. Washington, DC: National Highway Traffic Safety Association. http://www.nhtsa.gov.

92. National Highway Traffic Safety Administration. Traffic Safety Performance (Core Outcomes) Measures for Mississippi. Washington, DC: U.S. Department of Transportation. http://www-nrd.nhtsa.dot.gov.

93. Mendes, E. Smoking Rates Remain Highest in Kentucky, Lowest in Utah. Gallup. Nov 17, 2011. http://www.gallup.com.

94. Tobacco Control State Highlights. Atlanta, GA: National Center for Chronic Disease Prevention and Health Promotion; 2013. http://www.cdc.gov.

95. Tobacco Use in Mississippi. Jackson, MS: Mississippi Office of Tobacco Control. http://www.msdh.ms.gov.

96. Tobacco Use in Mississippi. Jackson, MS: Mississippi Office of Tobacco Control. http://www.msdh.ms.gov.

97. Burnett LE, Hoffman A. *Black is the new green: Marketing to affluent African Americans.* New York: Palgrave McMillan; 2010.

98. Williams DR, Jackson PB. Social Sources Of Racial Disparities In Health. *Health Affairs.* 2005;24(2):325-34.

99. Jackson DR, Williams PB. Social Sources of Racial Disparities. *Health Affairs.* 2005;24(2):325-334.

100. Smoking and Tobacco Control. Chapter 3 - Smoking Prevalence and Lung Cancer Death *Rates.* Rockville, MD: US National Institutes of Health; 2008. http:// www.cancer.gov.

101. Research and Program Services Epidemiology and Statistics Unit. Trends in Tobacco Use. Washington, DC: The American Lung Association; 2011. http:// www.lung.org.

102. Smoking prevalence and lung cancer deaths. chapter 3. http://cancercontrol.cancer.gov.

103. Clinical guidelines on the identification, evaluation, and treatment of overweight and obesity in adults. Bethesda, MD: National Institute of Health. http:// www.nhlbi.nih.gov.

104. Richie W. Blacks & Obesity: What are today's statistics? Washington, D.C.: Trust for America's Health. http://www.healthyamericans.org.

105. Levi J, Segal LM, St Laurent R, et al. *F as in Fat: How obesity threatens America's future.* Washington, DC: Trust for America's Health; 2012. http:// www.healthyamericans.org.

106. Rahman M, Berenson AB. Self-perception of weight and its association with weight-related behaviors in young, reproductive-aged women. *Obstet Gynecol. 2010;116(6):1274-80.* http://www.ncbi.nlm.nih.gov.

107. Black women & diabetes – More than a little sugar. Washington, DC: Black Women's Health Imperative. http://www. healthyblackwomen.org.

108. Norris M. *Why black women, infants lag in birth outcomes.* All Things Considered. Washington, DC: NPR. July 2011. http://www.npr.org.

109. Satpathy HK, Fleming A, Frey D, Barsoom M, Satpathy C, Khandalavala J. Maternal obesity and pregnancy. *Postgrad Med.* 2008;120(3):E01-9. http://www.ncbi.nlm.nih.gov.

110. Births:final data for 2010. table I–7 cesarean delivery, by race and Hispanic origin of mother: U.S., each state and territory, National Vital Statistics Reports.2010. Centers for Disease Control and Prevention. 2012; 61(1) p 11. http:// www.cdc.gov.

111. Stothard KJ, Tennant PW, Bell R, Rankin J. Maternal overweight and obesity and the risk of congenital anomalies: a systematic review and meta-analysis. *JAMA.* 2009 11;301(6):636-50. http://www.ncbi.nlm.nih.gov.

112. Anderson JL, Waller DK, Canfield MA, Shaw GM, Watkins ML, Werler MM. Maternal obesity, gestational diabetes, and central nervous system birth defects. *Epidemiology.* 2005;16(1):87-92. http://www.ncbi.nlm.nih.gov.

113. Unnatural Causes: When the Bough Breaks. PBS. Washington, DC: National Minority Consortium; 2008. http://www.npr.org.

114. Ogden CL, Lamb MM, Caroll MD, Flegal KM. *Obesity and socioeconomic status in adults: United States 2005-2008.* Hyattsville, MD: National Center for Health Statistics. Centers for Disease Control and Prevention; 2010. http://www.cdc.gov.

115. Ogden CL, Lamb MM, Carroll MD. Flegal KM. *Obesity and socioeconomic status in adults: US 2005 - 2008.* Hyattsville, MD: National Center of Health Statistics. Centers for Disease Control and Prevention; 2010. http://www.cdc.gov.

116. Ogden CL, Lamb MM, Caroll MD, Flegal KM. *Obesity and socioeconomic status in adults: U.S. 2005 - 2008.* Hyattsville, MD: National Center of Health Statistics. Centers for Disease Control and Prevention; 2010. http://www.cdc.gov.

117. Ogden CL, Lamb MM, Carroll MD, Flegal KM. *Obesity and Socioeconomic Status in Adults: U.S. 2005 - 2008.* Hyattsville, MD: National Center of Health Statistics. Centers for Disease Control and Prevention; 2010. http://www.cdc.gov.

118. Johnson-Taylor WL, Fishe RAr, Hubbard VS, Starke-Reed P, Eggers PS. The change in weight perception of weight status among the overweight: comparison of NHANES III (1988–1994) and 1999-2004 NHANES. *Int J Behav Nutr Phys Act.* 2008 12;5:9. http://www.ncbi.nlm.nih.gov.

119. Krauss RC, Powell LM, Wada R. Weight misperceptions and racial and ethnic disparities in adolescent female body mass index. *J Obes.* 2012;2012:205393. http://www.ncbi.nlm.nih.gov.

120. Rahman M, Berenson AB. Self-perception of weight and its association with weight-related behaviors in young, reproductive-aged women. *Obstet Gynecol.* 2010;116(6):1274-80. http://www.ncbi.nlm.nih.gov.

121. Hendley Y, Zhao L, Coverson DL, et al. Differences in weight perception among blacks and whites. *J Womens Health (Larchmt).* 2011;20(12):1805:11. http://www.ncbi.nlm.nih.gov.

122. Krauss RC, Powell LM, Wada R. Weight misperceptions and racial and ethnic disparities in adolescent female body mass index. *J Obes.* 2012;2012:205393. http://www.ncbi.nlm.nih.gov.

123. Thomas Am, Moseley G, Stallings R, Nichols-English G, Wagner PJ. Perceptions of Obesity: Black and White differences. *J Cult Divers.* 2008;15(4):174-80. http://www.ncbi.nlm.nih.gov.

124. Kleinrock M. *The Use of Medicines in the US: Review of 2011.* Parsippany, NJ: IMS Institute for Healtcare Informatics; 2012. http:// www.theimsinstitute.org.

125. Cox ER, Halloran DR., Homan SM, Welliver L, Mager DE. *Trends in the Prevalence of Chronic Medication Use in Children: 2002-2005.* 2008;122(5):e1053-61. http://www.ncbi.nlm.nih.gov.

126. FAERS Patient Outcomes by Year. Silver Spring, MD: U.S. Food and Drug Administration;2013. http://www.fda.gov.

127. Shepherd G, Mohorn P, Yacoub K, May DW. Adverse drug reaction deaths reported in United States vital statistics, 1999-2006. *Ann Pharmacother.* 2012;46(2):169-75. http://www.ncbi.nlm.nih.gov.

128. *Safer medicines for c hildren: The need to renew pediatric drug testing laws.* Washington, DC: American Academy of Pediatrics; 2007. http://www.aap.org.

129. Abel GA, Penson RT, Joffe S, et al. Direct-to-consumer advertising in oncology. *Oncologist.* 2006;11(2):217–226. http://www.ncbi.nlm.nih.gov.

130. DTC marketing mix: Radio and outdoor ad spending soars, Internet not so much. Pharma Marketing. *http://pharmamkting.blogspot.com/2010/06/dtc-marketing-mix-radio-outdoor-ad.html.*

131. Greene JA, Herzberg D. Hidden in plain sight: Marketing prescription drugs to consumers in the twentieth century. Am J Public Health. 2010;100(5):793–803. http://www.ncbi.nlm.nih.gov.

132. Ventola, CL. Direct-to-consumer pharmaceutical Advertising: Therapeutic or toxic? *P T. 2011;* 36(10): 669-674, 681-684. http://www.ncbi.nlm.nih.gov.

133. The impact ofdirect-to-consumer drug advertising on seniors' health and health care costs. Senate Special Committee on Aging. First Session ed. Washington, DC: US Government Printing Office; 2005.

134. Frosch DL, Krueger PM, Hornik RC, Cronholm PF, Barg FK. Creating demand for prescription drugs: a content analysis of television direct-to-consumer advertising. *Ann Fam Med.* 2007;5(1):6-13. http://www.ncbi.nlm.nih.gov.

135. Lo B, Field MJ. Conflict of Interest in Medical Research, Education, and Practice. Washington, DC: National Academies Press (US); 2009.

136. Relman, AS. *Your Doctor's Drug Problem.* New York, NY : New York Times, Nov 18 2003.

137. Weber T, Orstein C. Med Schools Flunk at Keeping Faculty Off Pharma Speaking Circuit. New York, NY: ProPublica; 2010. http://www.propublica.org.

138. Open Payments. Baltimore, MD: Centers for Medicare and Medicaid Services; 2013. http://www.cms.gov.

139. Eaton CB, Goodwin MA, Stange KC. Direct observation of nutrition counseling in family practice. *Am J Prev Med.* 2002;23(3):174-9.

140. Committee on Nutrition in Medical Education. Nutrition education in U.S. medical schools. Washington, DC: National Academy Press; 1985. http://www.nap.edu.

141. Frantz DJ, Munroe C, McClave SA, Martindale R. Current perception of nutrition education in U.S. medical schools. *Curr Gastroenterol Rep.* 2011;13(4):376-9. http://www.ncbi.nlm.nih.gov.

142. Adams KM, Lindell KC, Kohlmeier M, Zeisel SH. Status of nutrition education in medical schools. *Am J Clin Nutr.* 2006;83(4):941S-944S. http://www.ncbi.nlm.nih.gov.

143. Adams KM, Kohlmeier M, Zeisel SH. Nutrition Education in U.S. Medical Schools: Latest Update of a National Survey. *Acad Med.* 2010;85(9):1537-42. http://www.ncbi.nlm.nih.gov.

144. Dietary Supplements. Washington:DC FDA;2014.http://www.fda.gov.

145. Nutritional and dietary supplements long term contributions and lobbying, 2012 and Pharmaceutical manufacturing long term contributions and lobbying, 2013. Washington, DC: Center for Responsive Politics; 2013. http://www.opensecrets.org.

146. Dooling R. Health Care's Generation Gap. The New York Times [New York] August 16, 2009. http://www.nytimes.org.

147. Fisher ES, Wennberg DE, Stukel TA, Gottlieb DJ, Lucas FL, Pinder EL. The implications of regional variations in Medicare spending. Part 1: the content, quality, and accessibility of care. *Ann Intern Med.* 2003;138(4):273-87.

148. Fisher ES, Wennberg DE, Stukel TA, Gottlieb DJ, Lucas FL, Pinder EL.The implications of regional variations in Medicare spending. Part 2: health outcomes and satisfaction with care. *Ann Intern Med. 2003*;138(4):288-98.

149. Fisher E. More care is not better care. Washington, DC: NICHM Foundation; 2005. http:// www.nihcm.org.

150. Anderson G.Herbert R, Zeffiro T, Johnson N. Chronic conditions: making the case for ongoing care. Baltimore, MD: John Hopkins University; 2004. http://www.partnershipforsolution.org.

151. Levi J, Segal LM, Juliano C. Prevention for a healthier america:investments in disease prevention yield significant savings, stronger communities. Washington, DC:Trust for America's Health; 2008. http://healthyamericans.org/reports/prevention08.

152. Trust for America's Health. Key Health Data About Mississippi. Washingrton, DC; 2013. http://www.healthyamericans.org.

153. *FY 2013 Mississippi State Health Planel.* Jackson, MS: Mississippi State Department of Health; 2013. http://www.msdh.ms.gov.

154. Mississippi State Board of Health. Jackson, MS. State of Mississippi; 2013. http://www.msdh.ms.gov.

155. National prevention council action plan. Washington, DC: U.S. Surgeon General. National Prevention Council; 2012. http://www.surgeongeneral.gov.

156. Patient protection and affordable care act (HR 3590). Selected Prevention, Public Health & Workforce Provisions. Washington, DC; 2009. Trust for America's Health; 2009. http:// healthyamericans.org.

157. How the Health Care Law is Making a Difference for the People of Mississippi . Washington, DC: US Department of Health and Human Services; 2013. http://www.hhs.gov.

158. Knip M, Simell O. Environmental triggers of type 1 diabetes. *Cold Spring Harb Perspect Med.* 2012;2(7):a007690. http://www.ncbi.nlm.nih.gov.

159. Borch-Johnsen K, et al. Relation between breast-feeding and incidence rates of insulin-dependent diabetes mellitus. A hypothesis. *Lancet.* 1984;2(8411):1083-6. http://www.ncbi.nlm.nih.gov.

160. Dosch HM, Becker DJ. Infant feeding and autoimmune diabetes. *Adv Exp Med Biol.* 2002;503:133-40. http://www.ncbi.nlm.nih.gov.

161. Patelarou E, Girvalaki C, Brokalaki H, Patelarou A, Androulaki Z, Vardavas C. Current evidence on the associations of breastfeeding, infant formula, and cow's milk introduction with type 1 diabetes mellitus: a systematic review. *Nutr Rev.* 2012;70(9):509-19. http://www.ncbi.nlm.nih.gov.

162. Alves JG, Figueiroa JN, Meneses J, Alves GV. Breastfeeding protects against type 1 diabetes mellitus: a case-sibling study. *Breastfeed Med.* 2012;7(1):25-8. http://www.ncbi.nlm.nih.gov.

163. Mayer EJ, Hamman RF, Gay EC, Lezotte DC, Savitz DA, Klingensmith GJ. Reduced risk of IDDM among breast-fed children. The Colorado IDDM Registry. *Diabetes.* 1988;37(12):1625-32.

164. Virtanen SM, Räsänen L, Aro A, Ylönen K, Lounamaa R, Tuomilehto J, Akerblom HK. Feeding in infancy and the risk of type 1 diabetes mellitus in Finnish children. The 'Childhood Diabetes in Finland' Study Group. *Diabet Med.* 1992(9):815-9. http://www.ncbi.nlm.nih.gov.

165. Pettitt DJ, Forman MR, Hanson RL, Knowler WC, Bennett PH. Breastfeeding and incidence of non-insulin-dependent diabetes mellitus in Pima Indians. *Lancet.* 1997 Jul 19;350(9072):166-8. http://www.ncbi.nlm.nih.gov.

166. Virtanen SM, Räsänen L, Ylönen K, Aro A, Clayton D, Langholz B, Pitkäniemi J, Savilahti E, Lounamaa R, Tuomilehto J, et al. Early introduction of dairy products associated with increased risk of IDDM in Finnish children. The Childhood in Diabetes in Finland Study Group. *Diabetes.* 1993 Dec;42(12):1786-90. http://www.ncbi.nlm.nih.gov.

167. Sadauskaite-Kuehne V, Ludvigsson J, Padaiga Z, Jasinskiene E, Samuelsson U. Longer breastfeeding is an independent protective factor against development of type 1 diabetes mellitus in childhood. *Diabetes Metab Res Rev.* 2004;20(2):150-7.

168. Virtanen SM, Räsänen L, Aro A, Lindström J, Sippola H, Lounamaa R, Toivanen L, Tuomilehto J, Akerblom HK. Infant feeding in Finnish children less than 7 yr of age with newly diagnosed IDDM. Childhood Diabetes in Finland Study Group. *Diabetes Care.* 1991 May;14(5):415-7.

169. Riordan J, Auerbach KG. *Breastfeed and Human Lactation 2nd Edition.* Sudbury, MA: Jones and Bartlett Publishers; 1998.

170. Silfverdal SA, Bodin L, Ulanova M, Hahn-Zoric M, Hanson LA, Olcén P. Expression of idiotypic antibodies-1 and -2 and breastfeeding in relation to antibody levels against Haemophilus influenzae type B in children. *Scand J Immunol.* 2006;63(5):371-5. http://www.ncbi.nlm.nih.gov.

171. Melendi GA, Coviello S, Bhat N, Zea-Hernandez J, Ferolla FM, Polack FP. Breastfeeding is associated with the production of type I interferon in infants infected with influenza virus. *Acta Paediatr. 2010 Oct;99(10):1517-21.* http://www.ncbi.nlm.nih.gov.

172. Chantry CJ, Howard CR, Auinger P. Full breastfeeding duration and associated decrease in respiratory tract infection in US children. *Pediatrics.* 2006;117(2):425-32. http://www.ncbi.nlm.nih.gov.

173. Chantry CJ, Howard CR, Auinger P. Full breastfeeding duration and associated decrease in respiratory tract infection in US children. *Pediatrics.* 2006;117(2):425-32. http://www.ncbi.nlm.nih.gov.

174. Golding J, Emmett PM, Rogers IS. Does breast feeding protect against nongastric infections? *Early Hum Dev. 1997* 29;49 Suppl:S105-20. http://www.ncbi.nlm.nih.gov.

175. Okamoto Y, Tsutsumi H, Kumar NS, Ogra PL. Effect of breast feeding on the development of anti-idiotype antibody response to F glycoprotein of respiratory syncytial virus in infant mice after post-partum maternal immunization. J Immunol. 1989;142(7):2507-12. http://www.ncbi.nlm.nih.gov.

176. Nishimura T, Suzue J, Kaji H. Breastfeeding reduces the severity of respiratory syncytial virus infection among young infants: a multi-center prospective study. *Pediatr Int.* 2009;51(6):812-6. http://www.ncbi.nlm.nih.gov.

177. Bryan DL, Hart PH, Forsyth KD, Gibson RA. Immunomodulatory constituents of human milk change in response to infant bronchiolitis. *Pediatr Allergy Immunol.* 2007;18(6):495-502.

178. Roine I, Fernandez JA, Vásquez A, Cáneo M. Breastfeeding reduces immune activation in primary respiratory syncytial virus infection. *Eur Cytokine Netw.* 2005;16(3):206-10. http://www.ncbi.nlm.nih.gov.

179. Sinha A, Madden J, Ross-Degnan D, Soumerai S, Platt R. Reduced risk of neonatal respiratory infections among breastfed girls but not boys. *Pediatrics.* 2003;112(4):e303. http://www.ncbi.nlm.nih.gov.

180. Chiba Y, Minagawa T, Mito K, et al. Effect of breast feeding on responses of systemic interferon and virus-specific lymphocyte transformation in infants with respiratory syncytial virus infection. *J Med Virol.* 1987;21(1):7-14. http://www.ncbi.nlm.nih.gov.

181. Pisacane A, Graziano L, Mazzarella G, et al. Breast-feeding and urinary tract infection. *J Pediatr.* 1992;120:87–89. http://www.ncbi.nlm.nih.gov.

182. Beaudry M, Dufour R, Marcoux S. Relation between infant feeding and infections during the first six months of life. *J Pediatr.* 1995;126:191–197. http://www.ncbi.nlm.nih.gov.

183. Kramer MS, Kakuma R. Optimal duration of exclusive breastfeeding. *Cochrane Database Syst Rev.* 2012;8:CD003517. http://www.ncbi.nlm.nih.gov.

184. Aguiar H, Silva AI. Breastfeeding: the importance of intervening. *Acta Med Port.* 2011;24 Suppl 4:889-96. http://www.ncbi.nlm.nih.gov.

185. Silfverdal SA, Bodin L, Olcén P. Protective effect of breastfeeding: an ecologic study of Haemophilus influenzae meningitis and breastfeeding in a Swedish population. *Int J Epidemiol.* 1999;28(1):152-6. http://www.ncbi.nlm.nih.gov.

186. Gessner BD, Ussery XT, Parkinson AJ, Breiman RF. Risk factors for invasive disease caused by Streptococcus pneumoniae among Alaska native children younger than two years of age. *Pediatr Infect Dis J.* 1995;14(2):123-8. http://www.ncbi.nlm.nih.gov.

187. Ford RPK, Taylor BJ, Mitchell EA, et al. Breastfeeding and the risk of sudden infant death syndrome. *Int J Epidemiol.* 1993;22:885–890. http://www.ncbi.nlm.nih.gov.

188. Aguiar H, Silva AI. Breastfeeding: the importance of intervening. *Acta Med Port. 2011;24 Suppl 4:889-96.* http://www.ncbi.nlm.nih.gov.

189. Koletzko S, Sherman P, Corey M, Griffiths A, Smith C. Role of infant feeding practices in development of Crohn's disease in childhood. *BMJ.* 1989;298(6688):1617-8. http://www.ncbi.nlm.nih.gov.

190. Rigas A, et al. Breast-feeding and maternal smoking in the etiology of Crohn's disease and ulcerative colitis in childhood. *Ann Epidemiol.* 1993;3(4):387-92. http://www.ncbi.nlm.nih.gov. http://www.ncbi.nlm.nih.gov.

191. Henriksson C, Boström AM, Wiklund IE. What effect does breastfeeding have on coeliac disease? A systematic review update. *Evid Based Med.* 2013;18(3):98-103. http://www.ncbi.nlm.nih.gov.

192. Bouguerra F, Hajjem S, Guilloud-Bataille M, Khlat M, Khaldi F, Bennaceur B. [Breast feeding effect relative to age of onset of celiac disease]. *Arch Pediatr.* 1998;5(6):621-6. http://www.ncbi.nlm.nih.gov.

193. Bener A, Hoffmann GF, Afify Z, Rasul K, Tewfik I. Does prolonged breastfeeding reduce the risk for childhood leukemia and lymphomas? *Minerva Pediatr.* 2008;60(2):155-61. http://www.ncbi.nlm.nih.gov.

194. Kwan ML, Buffler PA, Abrams B, Kiley VA. Breastfeeding and the risk of childhood leukemia: a meta-analysis. *Public Health Rep.* 2004;119(6):521-35. http://www.ncbi.nlm.nih.gov.

195. Rigas A, Rigas B, Glassman M, Yen YY, Lan SJ, Petridou E, Hsieh CC, Trichopoulos D. Breast-feeding and maternal smoking in the etiology of Crohn's disease and ulcerative colitis in childhood. *Ann Epidemiol.* 1993;3(4):387-92. http://www.ncbi.nlm.nih.gov.

196. Dewey KG, Heinig MJ, Nommsen-Rivers LA. Differences in morbidity between breast-fed and formula-fed infants. *J Pediatr.* 1995;126:696–702. http://www.ncbi.nlm.nih.gov.

197. Das JK, Salam RA, Bhutta ZA. Global burden of childhood diarrhea and interventions. *Curr Opin Infect Dis.* 2014;27(5):451-8.

198. Riordan J, Auerbach KG. *Breastfeeding and Human Lactation 2nd Edition.* Sudbury, MA:Jones and Bartlett;1998:141.

199. Turner JR. Intestinal mucosal barrier function in health and disease. *Nat Rev Immunol.* 2009;9(11):799-809. http://www.ncbi.nlm.nih.gov.

200. Riordan J, Auerbach. *Breastfeeding and Human Lactation 2nd edition.* Sudbury, MA : Jones and Bartlett Publishers, 1998.

201. Xanthou M, Bines J, Walker WA. Human milk and intestinal host defense in newborns: an update. *Adv Pediatr.* 1995;42:171-208. http://www.ncbi.nlm.nih.gov.

202. Turner JR. Intestinal mucosal barrier function in health and disease. *Nat Rev Immunol.* 2009;9(11):799-809. http://www.ncbi.nlm.nih.gov.

203. Sekirov I, Russell SL, Caetano L, Antunes CM, Finlay BB. Gut microbiota in health and disease. *Physiol Rev.*2010;90(3): 859-904. http://www.ncbi.nlm.nih.gov.

204. Riordan J, Auerbach KG. *Breastfeeding and Human Lactation 2nd Edition.* Sudbury, MA:Jones and Bartlett;1998:142-145.

205. Weaver WT, Arthur H, Bunn J, Thomas JE. Human milk IgA concentrations during the first year of lactation. *Arch Dis Child.* 1998;78:235-239. http://www.ncbi.nlm.nih.gov.

206. Hanson LA, Hahn-Zoric M, Berndes M, et al. Breast feeding: overview and breast milk immunology. *Acta Paediatr Jpn.* 1994;36(5):557-61. http://www.ncbi.nlm.nih.gov.

207. Hanson LA, Söderström T. Human milk: Defense against infection. *Prog Clin Biol Res.* 1981;61:147-59. http://www.ncbi.nlm.nih.gov.

208. Noguera-Obenza M, Ochoa TJ, Gomez HF, et al. Human milk secretory antibodies against attaching and effacing Escherichia coli antigens. *Emerg Infect Dis.* 2003;9(5):545-51. http://www.ncbi.nlm.nih.gov.

209. Knip M, Simell O. Environmental triggers of type 1 diabetes. *Cold Spring Harb Perspect Med.* 2012;2(7):a007690. http://www.ncbi.nlm.nih.gov.

210. Ylipaasto P, Smura T, Gopalacharyulu P, et al. Enterovirus-induced gene expression profile is critical for human pancreatic islet destruction. *Diabetologia.* 2012;55(12):3273-83. http://www.ncbi.nlm.nih.gov.

211. Richardson SJ, Leete P, Bone AJ, Foulis AK, Morgan NG. Expression of the enteroviral capsid protein VP1 in the islet cells of patients with type 1 diabetes is associated with induction of protein kinase R and downregulation of Mcl-1. *Diabetologia.* 2013;56(1):185-93. http://www.ncbi.nlm.nih.gov.

212. Rešić Lindehammer S, Honkanen H, Nix WA, Oikarinen M, et al. Seroconversion to islet autoantibodies after enterovirus infection in early pregnancy. *Viral Immunol. 2012;25(4):254-61.* http://www.ncbi.nlm.nih.gov.

213. Hyoty H. Enterovirus infections and type 1 diabetes. *Ann Med.*2002; 34:138–47. http://www.ncbi.nlm.nih.gov.

214. Oikarinen M, Tauriainen S, Honkanen T, et al. Detection of enteroviruses in the intestine of type 1 diabetic patients. *Clin Exp Immunol.* 2008;151(1):71-5. http://www.ncbi.nlm.nih.gov.

215. Riordan J, Auerbach KG. *Breastfeeding and Human Lactation* 2nd Edition. Sudbury, MA:Jones and Bartlett Publishers;1988:147.

216. Bainter B. *Intestinal Absorption of Macromolecules and Immune Transmission from Mother to Young.* CRC Press: Boca Raton, FL,1986; p107.

217. Riordan J, Auerbach KG. *Breastfeeding and Human Lactation* 2nd Edition. Sudsbury, MA:Jones and Bartlett Publishers; 1988:147.

218. Harrison LC, Honeyman MC. Cow's milk and type 1 diabetes: the real debate is about mucosal immune function. *Diabetes.*1999;48:1501–1507. http://www.ncbi.nlm.nih.gov.

219. Knip M, Simell O. Environmental Triggers and Type 1 Diabetes. *Cold Spring Harb Perspect Med. 2012;2(7):a007690.* http://www.ncbi.nlm.nih.gov.

220. Virtanen SM, Aro A, Clayton D. et al. Early Introduction of Dairy Products Associated with Increased Risk of IDDM in Finnish Children. *Diabetes.1993;42(12):1786-1790.* http://www.ncbi.nlm.nih.gov.

221. Gimeno SG, de Souza JM. IDDM and milk consumption. A case-control study in São Paulo, Brazil. *Diabetes Care.* 1997;20(8):1256-60. http://www.ncbi.nlm.nih.gov.

222. Gerstein HC. The relationship between cow's milk exposure and Type 1 Diabetes. *Diabetes Med.* 1997;13(1):23-9. http://www.ncbi.nlm.nih.gov.

223. Strotmeyer ES, Yang Z, LaPorte RE, et al. Infant diet and type 1 diabetes in China. *Diabetes Res Clin Pract.* 2004;65(3):283-92. http://www.ncbi.nlm.nih.gov.

224. Virtanen SM, Räsänen L, Aro A,. Infant feeding in Finnish children less than 7 yr of age with newly diagnosed IDDM. Childhood Diabetes in Finland Study Group. *Diabetes Care.* 1991;14(5):415-7. http://www.ncbi.nlm.nih.gov.

225. Rosenbauer J, Herzig P, Kaiser P, Giani G. Early nutrition and risk of Type 1 diabetes mellitus--a nationwide case-control study in preschool children. *Exp Clin Endocrinol Diabetes.* 2007;115(8):502-8. http://www.ncbi.nlm.nih.gov.

226. Pérez-Bravo F, Oyarzún A, Carrasco E, Albala C, Dorman JS, Santos JL. Duration of breast feeding and bovine serum albumin antibody levels in type 1 diabetes: a case-control study. *Pediatr Diabetes.* 2003;4(4):157-61. http://www.ncbi.nlm.nih.gov.

227. Karjalainen J, Martin JM, Knip M, et al. A bovine albumin peptide as a possible trigger of insulin-dependent diabetes mellitus. *N Engl J Med.* 1992;327(5):302-7. http://www.ncbi.nlm.nih.gov.

228. Dahlquist G, Savilahti E, Landin-Olsson M. An increased level of antibodies to beta-lactoglobulin is a risk determinant for early-onset type 1 (insulin-dependent) diabetes mellitus independent of islet cell antibodies and early introduction of cow's milk. *Diabetologia.* 1992;35(10):980-4. http://www.ncbi.nlm.nih.gov.

229. Savilahti E, Akerblom HK, Tainio VM, Koskimies S. Children with newly diagnosed insulin dependent diabetes mellitus have increased levels of cow's milk antibodies. *Diabetes Res.* 1988;7(3):137-40. http://www.ncbi.nlm.nih.gov.

230. Saukkonen T, Savilahti E, Madácsy L, et al. Increased frequency of IgM antibodies to cow's milk proteins in Hungarian children with newly diagnosed insulin-dependent diabetes mellitus. *Eur J Pediatr.* 1996;155(10):885-9. http://www.ncbi.nlm.nih.gov.

231. Vähäsalo P, Petäys T, Knip M, et al. Relation between antibodies to islet cell antigens, other autoantigens and cow's milk proteins in diabetic children and unaffected siblings at the clinical manifestation of IDDM. The Childhood Diabetes in Finland Study Group. *Autoimmunity.* 1996;23(3):165-74. http://www.ncbi.nlm.nih.gov.

232. Vaarala O, Knip M, Paronen J, et al. Cow's milk feeding induces primary immunization to insulin in infants at genetic risk for type 1 diabetes. *Diabetes.* 1999;48(7):1389-94. http://www.ncbi.nlm.nih.gov.

233. Karppinen M, et al. Significance of cow's milk protein antibodies as risk factor for childhood IDDM: interactions with dietary cow's milk intake and HLA-DQB1 genotype. Childhood Diabetes in Finland Study Group. Diabetologia. 1998;41(1):72-8.

234. Savilahti E, Saukkonen TT, Virtala ET, Tuomilehto J, Akerblom HK. Increased levels of cow's milk and beta-lactoglobulin antibodies in young children with newly diagnosed IDDM. The Childhood Diabetes in Finland Study Group. *Diabetes Care.* 1993;16(7):984-9. http://www.ncbi.nlm.nih.gov.

235. Virtanen SM, Saukkonen T, Savilahti E, et al. Diet, cow's milk protein antibodies and the risk of IDDM in Finnish children. Childhood Diabetes in Finland Study Group. *Diabetologia.* 1994;37(4):381-7. http://www.ncbi.nlm.nih.gov.

236. Saukkonen T, Virtanen SM, Karppinen M, et al. Significance of cow's milk protein antibodies as risk factor for childhood IDDM: interactions with dietary cow's milk intake and HLA-DQB1 genotype. Childhood Diabetes in Finland Study Group. Diabetologia.1998;41(1):72-8

237. Neyestani TR, Djalali M, Pezeshki M, et al. Serum antibodies to the major proteins found in cow's milk of Iranian patients with Type 1 diabetes mellitus. Diabetes Nutr Metab. 2004;17(2):76-83.

238. Work Group on Cow's Milk Protein and Diabetes Mellitus. Infant Feeding Practices and Their Possible Relationship to the Etiology of Diabetes Mellitus. *Pediatrics* 1994; 94:752-754. http://www.ncbi.nlm.nih.gov.

239. Gillman MW. First months of life: a critical period for development of obesity. *Am J Clin Nutr.* 2008;87(6):1587–1589. http://www.ncbi.nlm.nih.gov.

240. Stettler N, Zemel BS, Kumanyika S, Stallings VA. Infant weight gain and childhood overweight status in multicenter, cohort study. *Pediatrics.* 2002;109(2):194–199. http://www.ncbi.nlm.nih.gov.

241. Ong KK. Size at birth, postnatal growth and risk of obesity. *Horm Res.* 2006;65 (suppl 3) 65- 69. http://www.ncbi.nlm.nih.gov.

242. Dietz WH. Overweight and precursors of type 2 diabetes mellitus in children and adolescents. *J Pediatr* 2001;138 (4) 453-454. http://www.ncbi.nlm.nih.gov.

243. Must A, Spadano J, Coakley EH, Field AE, Colditz G, Dietz WH. The disease burden associated with overweight and obesity. *JAMA 1999;*282 (16) 1523-1529. http://www.ncbi.nlm.nih.gov.

244. Report of the expert consultation on the optimal duration of exclusive breastfeeding. Geneva, Switzerland: World Health Organization; 2001.

245. Pediatric Nutrition Handbook. 6th ed. Elk Grove Village, IL: American Academy of Pediatrics; 2009.

246. Breastfeeding and the Use of Human Milk. *Pediatrics.*2005;115(2): 496-506. http://www.ncbi.nlm.nih.gov.

247. Huh SY, Rifas-Shiman SL, Taveras EM, Oken E, Gillman MW. Timing of Solid Food Introduction and Risk of Obesity in Preschool-Aged Children. *Pediatrics.* 2011;127(3):e544-51. http://www.ncbi.nlm.nih.gov.

248. Baker JL, Michaelsen KF, Rasmussen KM, Sorensen TI. Maternal prepregnant body mass index, duration of breastfeeding, and timing of complementary food introduction are associated with infant weight gain. *Am J Clin Nutr.* 2004;80(6):1579–1588. http://www.ncbi.nlm.nih.gov.

249. Kostraba JN, Cruickshanks KJ, Lawler-Heavner J, et al. *Early exposure to cow's milk and solid foods in infancy, genetic predisposition, and risk of IDDM.* Diabetes. 1993;42(2):288-95. http://www.ncbi.nlm.nih.gov.

250. Norris JM, Barriga K, Klingensmith G, et al.. Timing of initial cereal exposure in infancy and risk of islet autoimmunity. *JAMA.* 2003;290(13):1713-20. http://www.ncbi.nlm.nih.gov.

251. Ziegler AG, Schmid S, Huber D, Hummel M, Bonifacio E. Early infant feeding and risk of developing type 1 diabetes-associated autoantibodies. *JAMA.* 2003;290(13):1721-8. http://www.ncbi.nlm.nih.gov.

252. Snell-Bergeon JK, Smith J, Dong F, Barón AE, Barriga K, Norris JM, Rewers M. Early childhood infections and the risk of islet autoimmunity: the Diabetes Autoimmunity Study in the Young (DAISY). Diabetes Care. 2012;35(12):2553-8. http://www.ncbi.nlm.nih.gov.

253. Guandalini S. The influence of gluten: weaning recommendations for healthy children and children at risk for celiac disease. *Nestle Nutr Workshop Ser Pediatr Program. 2007;*60:139-51; discussion 151-5.

254. Bouguerra F, Hajjem S, Guilloud-Bataille M, Khlat M, Khaldi F, Bennaceur B. Breast feeding effect relative to age of onset of celiac disease. *Arch Pediatr.*1998;5(6):621-6. http://www.ncbi.nlm.nih.gov.

255. Sekirov I, Russell SL, Antunes CM, Finlay BB. Gut Microbiota in Health and Disease. *Physiol Rev.*2010;90(3): 859-904. http://www.ncbi.nlm.nih.gov.

256. Azad MB, et al. Gut microbiota of healthy Canadian infants:profiles by mode of delivery and infant diet at 4 months. *CMAJ.* 2013.19;185(5):385-94.

257. Ray K. Gut microbiota: Married to our gut microbiota. *Nat Rev Gastroenterol Hepatol.* 2012;9(10):555. http://www.ncbi.nlm.nih.gov.

258. Huurre A, Kalliomaki M, Rautava S, Rinne M, Salminen S, Isolauri E. Mode of delivery - effects on gut microbiota and humoral immunity. *Neonatology.* 2008;93(4):236-40. http://www.ncbi.nlm.nih.gov.

259. Ostfeld E, Segal J, Segal A, Bogokovski B. Bacterial colonization of the nose and external ear canal in newborn infants. *Isr J Med Sci.* 1983;19(12):1046-9. http://www.ncbi.nlm.nih.gov.

260. Biasucci G, Rubini M, Riboni S, Morelli L, Bessi E, Retetangos C. Mode of delivery affects the bacterial community in the newborn gut. *Early Hum Dev.* 2010;86 Suppl 1:13-5. http://www.ncbi.nlm.nih.gov.

261. Sekirov I, Russell SL, Antunes CM, Finlay BB. Gut Microbiota in Health and Disease. *Physiol Rev.*2010;90(3): 859-904. http://www.ncbi.nlm.nih.gov.

262. Mandar R, mikelsaar M. Transmission of mother's microflora to the newborn at birth. *Biol Neonate.1996; 69: 30–3.* http://www.ncbi.nlm.nih.gov.

263. Hegde S, Munshi AK. Influence of the maternal vaginal microbiota on the oral microbiota of the newborn. *J Clin Pediatr Dent.* 1998;22(4):317-21. http://www.ncbi.nlm.nih.gov.

264. Huurre A, Kalliomaki M, Rautava S, Rinne M, Salminen S, Isolauri E. Mode of delivery - effects on gut microbiota and humoral immunity. *Neonatology.* 2008;93(4):236-40. http://www.ncbi.nlm.nih.gov.

265. Dominguez-Bello MG, Costello EK, Contreras M, Magris M, Hidalgo G, Fierer N, Knight R. Delivery mode shapes the acquisition and structure of the initial microbiota across multiple body habitats in newborns. *Proc Natl Acad Sci U S A.* 2010;107(26):11971-5. http://www.ncbi.nlm.nih.gov.

266. Penders J, et al. Factors influencing the composition of the intestinal microbiota in early infancy. *Pediatrics.* 2006;118(2):511-21.

267. Phillips J, Gill N, Sikdar K, Penney S, Newhook LA. History of cesarean section associated with childhood onset of T1DM in Newfoundland and Labrador, Canada. *J Environ Public Health.* 2012;2012:635097. http://www.ncbi.nlm.nih.gov.

268. Cardwell CR, Stene LC, Joner G, et al. Caesarean section is associated with an increased risk of childhood-onset type 1 diabetes mellitus: a meta-analysis of observational studies. *Diabetologia.* 2008;51(5):726-35. http://www.ncbi.nlm.nih.gov.

269. Bonifacio E, Warncke K, Winkler C, Wallner M, Ziegler AG. Cesarean Section and Interferon-Induced Helicase Gene Polymorphisms Combine to Increase Childhood Type 1 Diabetes Risk. *Diabetes.* 2011; 60(12):3300–3306.

270. Thavagnanam S, Fleming J, Bromley A, Shields MD, Cardwell CR. A meta-analysis of the association between Caesarean section and childhood asthma. *Clin Exp Allergy.* 2008;38(4):629-33. http://www.ncbi.nlm.nih.gov.

271. Bager P, Wohlfahrt J, Westergaard T. Caesarean delivery and risk of atopy and allergic disease: meta-analyses. *Clin Exp Allergy.* 2008;38(4):634-42. http://www.ncbi.nlm.nih.gov.

272. Koplin J, Allen K, Gurrin L, Osborne N, Tang ML, Dharmage S. Is caesarean delivery associated with sensitization to food allergens and IgE-mediated food allergy: a systematic review. *Pediatr Allergy Immunol.* 2008;19(8):682-7. http://www.ncbi.nlm.nih.gov.

273. Renz-Polster H, David MR, Buist AS, Vollmer WM, O'Connor EA, Frazier EA, Wall MA. Caesarean section delivery and the risk of allergic disorders in childhood. *Clin Exp Allergy.* 2005;35(11):1466-72. http://www.ncbi.nlm.nih.gov.

274. Martin, JA Hamilton, BE, Ventura SJ, et al. Births: Final Data for 2011- National Vital *Statistics Reports.* Hyattsville, MD: National Vital Statistics Systems. National Center for Health Statistics. CDC; 2011.

275. Roth LM, Henley MM. Unequal Motherhood: Racial-Ethnic and Socioeconomic Disparities in Cesarean Sections in the United States. *Social Problems.* 2012;59[2]:207-227.

276. Menacker F, Hamilton BE. Recent Trends in Cesarean Delivery in the United States - NCH Data Brief No 35. Hyattsville, MD. U.S.: Health and Human Services. Center for Health Statistics.;2010. http://www.cdc.gov.

277. Linda LA. Cod liver oil, young children, and upper respiratory tract infections. *J Am Coll Nutr. 2010;29(6):559-62.* http://www.ncbi.nlm.nih.gov.

278. Stene LC, Joner G and Group, Norwegian Childhood Diabetes Study. Use of cod liver oil during the first year of life is associated with lower risk of childhood-onset type 1 diabetes: a large, population-based, case-control study. *Am J Clin Nutr.* 2003;78(6):1128-34.

279. Norris JM, Yin X, Lamb MM, et al. Omega-3 polyunsaturated fatty acid intake and islet autoimmunity in children at increased risk for type 1 diabetes. *JAMA.* 2007;298(12):1420-8.

280. Stene LC, Ulriksen J, Magnus P, Joner G. Use of cod liver oil during pregnancy associated with lower risk of Type I diabetes in the offspring. *Diabetologia.* 2000;43(9):1093-8. http://www.ncbi.nlm.nih.gov.

281. Fronczak CM, Baron AE, Chase HP, et al. In utero dietary exposures and risk of islet autoimmunity in children. *Diabetes Care.* 2003;26(12):3237-42. http://www.ncbi.nlm.nih.gov.

282. Hypponen E, Laara E, Reunanen A, Jarvelin MR, Virtanen SM. Intake of vitamin D and risk of type 1 diabetes: a birth-cohort study. *Lancet. 2001*;358(9292):1500-3. http://www.ncbi.nlm.nih.gov.

283. Littorin B, Blom P, Scholin A, et al. Lower levels of plasma 25-hydroxyvitamin D among young adults at diagnosis of autoimmune type 1 diabetes compared with control subjects: results from the nationwide Diabetes Incidence Study in Sweden (DISS). *Diabetologia.* 2006:49(12):2847-52.

284. Bener A, Alsaied A, Al-Ali M, et al. High prevalence of vitamin D deficiency in type 1 diabetes mellitus and healthy children.*Acta Diabetol.* 2009;46(3):183-9.

285. Riordan J, Auerbach KG. *Breastfeeding and Human Lactation 2nd Edition.* Spudbury,MA: Bartlett and Jones; 1998. http://www.ncbi.nlm.nih.gov.

286. Harder T, Bergmann R, Kallischnigg G, Plagemann A. Duration of breastfeeding and risk of overweight: a meta-analysis. *Am J Epidemiol.* 2005 1;162(5):397-403. http://www.ncbi.nlm.nih.gov.

287. Owen CG, Martin RM, Whincup PH, et al. Effect of infant feeding on the risk of obesity across the life course: a quantitative review of published evidence. *Pediatrics.* 2005;115:1367–1377. http://www.ncbi.nlm.nih.gov.

288. Arenz S, Rückerl R, Koletzko B, von Kries R. Breast-feeding and childhood obesity--a systematic review. *Int J Obes Relat Metab Disord.* 2004;28(10):1247-56. http://www.ncbi.nlm.nih.gov.

289. Ip S, Chung M, Raman G, et al. Breastfeeding and maternal and infant health outcomes in developed countries. *Evid Rep Technol Assess (Full Rep)* 2007;153:1–186. http://www.ncbi.nlm.nih.gov.

290. Horta BL, Bahl R, Martinés JC, et al. Evidence on the long-term effects of breastfeeding: systematic review and meta-analyses. Geneva, Switzerland: World Health Organization; 2007. pp. 1–57.

291. Dewey KG, Heinig MJ, Nommsen LA, Peerson JM, Lönnerdal B. Growth of breast-fed and formula-fed infants from 0 to 18 months: the DARLING Study. *Pediatrics.* 1992;89(6 Pt 1):1035-41. http://www.ncbi.nlm.nih.gov.

292. Riordan J, Auerbach KG. *Breastfeeding and Human Lactation 2nd Edition.* Spudbury,MA: Bartlett and Jones; 1998. http://www.ncbi.nlm.nih.gov.

293. Shu XO, Linet MS, Steinbuch M, et al. Breast-feeding and risk of childhood

acute leukemia. *J Natl Cancer Inst.* 1999;91(20):1765-72. http://www.ncbi.nlm.nih.gov.

294. Kwan ML, Buffler PA, Abrams B, Kiley VA. Breastfeeding and the risk of childhood leukemia: a meta-analysis. *Public Health Rep.* 2004;119(6):521-35. http://www.ncbi.nlm.nih.gov.

295. Altinkaynak S, Selimoglu MA, Turgut A, Kilicaslan B, Ertekin V. Breastfeeding duration and childhood acute leukemia and lymphomas in a sample of Turkish children. *J Pediatr Gastroenterol Nutr.* 2006;42(5):568-72. http://www.ncbi.nlm.nih.gov.

296. McNally RJ, Parker L. Environmental factors and childhood acute leukemias and lymphomas. *Leuk Lymphoma.* 2006;47(4):583-98. http://www.ncbi.nlm.nih.gov.

297. Guise JM, Austin D, Morris CD. Review of case-control studies related to breastfeeding and reduced risk of childhood leukemia. *Pediatrics.* 2005;116(5):e724-31. http://www.ncbi.nlm.nih.gov.

298. UK Childhood Cancer Study Investigators. Breastfeeding and childhood cancer. *Br J Cancer.* 2001;85(11):1685-94. http://www.ncbi.nlm.nih.gov.

299. Davis. MK. Review of the evidence for an association between infant feeding and childhood cancer. *Int J Cancer Suppl.* 1998;11:29-33. http://www.ncbi.nlm.nih.gov.

300. Martin RM, Gunnell D, Owen CG, Smith GD. Breast-feeding and childhood cancer: A systematic review with metaanalysis. *Int J Cancer.* 2005;117(6):1020-31. http://www.ncbi.nlm.nih.gov.

301. Hu FB. Globalization of diabetes: the role of diet, lifestyle, and genes. *Diabetes Care. 2011* Jun;34(6):1249-57. http://www.ncbi.nlm.nih.gov.

302. National Diabetes Fact Sheet: Diagnosed and undiagnosed diabetes in the United States, all ages. Atlanta, GA. Centers for Disease Control and Prevention; 2011. http://www.cdc.gov.

303. National Diabetes Fact Sheet. Diagnosed and undiagnosed diabetes in the United States, all ages. Atlanta, Georga. Centers for Disease Control and Prevention. http://www.cdc.gov.

304. Margolis DJ, Hoffstad O, Nafash J, Leonard CE, Freeman CP, Hennessy S, Wiebe DJ. Location, location, location: geographic clustering of lower-extremity amputation among Medicare beneficiaries with diabetes. *Diabetes Care. 2011;34(11):2363-7. http://www.ncbi.nlm.nih.gov.*

305. Kosaka K, Noda M, Kuzuya T. Prevention of type 2 diabetes by lifestyle intervention: a Japanese trial in IGT males. *Diabetes Res Clin Pract.* 2005;67(2):152-62. http://www.ncbi.nlm.nih.gov.

306. Orozco LJ, Buchleitner AM, Gimenez-Perez G, et al. Exercise or exercise and diet for preventing type 2 diabetes mellitus. *Cochrane Database Syst Rev.* 2008; 16;(3):CD003054. http://www.ncbi.nlm.nih.gov.

307. Schulze MB, Hu FB. Primary prevention of diabetes: what can be done and how much can be prevented? Annu Rev Public Health. 2005;26:445-67.

308. Astrup A. Healthy lifestyles in Europe: prevention of obesity and type II diabetes by diet and physical activity. *Public Health Nutr.* 2001;4(2B):499-515. http://www.ncbi.nlm.nih.gov.

309. Salas-Salvadó J, Martinez-González MÁ, Bulló M, Ros E. The role of diet in the prevention of type 2 diabetes. *Nutr Metab Cardiovasc Dis.* 2011;21 Suppl 2:B32-48. http://www.ncbi.nlm.nih.gov.

310. Hu FB. Diet, lifestyle, and the risk of type 2 diabetes mellitus in women. *N Engl J Med.* 2001;345(11):790-7. http://www.ncbi.nlm.nih.gov.

311. Tuomilehto J, et al. Prevention of type 2 diabetes mellitus by changes in lifestyle among subjects with impaired glucose tolerance. *N Engl J Med.* 2001;344(18):1343-50. http://www.ncbi.nlm.nih.gov.

312. Barnard RJ, Lattimore L, Holly RG, Cherny S, Pritikin N. Response of non-insulin-dependent diabetic patients to an intensive program of diet and exercise. Diabetes Care. 1982;5(4):370-4. http://www.ncbi.nlm.nih.gov.

313. Barnard RJ, Massey MR, Cherny S, O'Brien LT, Pritikin N. Long-term use of a high-complex-carbohydrate, high-fiber, low-fat diet and exercise in the treatment of NIDDM patients. http://www.ncbi.nlm.nih.gov.

314. Mishra S, Barnard ND, Gonzales J, Xu J, Agarwal U, Levin S. Nutrient intake in the GEICO multicenter trial: the effects of a multicomponent worksite intervention. *Eur J Clin Nutr.* 2013;67(10):1066-71. http://www.ncbi.nlm.nih.gov.

315. Jenkins DJ. Type 2 diabetes and the vegetarian diet. Am J Clin Nutr. 2003 Sep;78(3 Suppl):610S-616S. http://www.ncbi.nlm.nih.gov.

316. Trapp C, Barnard N, Katcher H. A plant-based diet for type 2 diabetes: scientific support and practical. strategies. Diabetes Educ. 2010;36(1):33-48. http://www.ncbi.nlm.nih.gov.

317. Barnard ND, Cohen J, Jenkins DJ, et al. A low-fat vegan diet improves glycemic control and cardiovascular risk factors in a randomized clinical trial in individuals with type 2 diabetes. *Diabetes Care.* 2006;29(8):1777-83. http://www.ncbi.nlm.nih.gov.

318. Barnard ND, Cohen J, Jenkins DJ, Turner-McGrievy G, Gloede L, Green A, Ferdowsian H. A low-fat vegan diet and a conventional diabetes diet in the treatment of type 2 diabetes: a randomized, controlled, 74-wk clinical trial. *Am J Clin Nutr.* 2009;89(5):1588S-1596S. http://www.ncbi.nlm.nih.gov.

319. Turner-McGrievy GM, Jenkins DJ, Barnard ND, Cohen J, Gloede L,

Green AA. Decreases in dietary glycemic index are related to weight loss among individuals following therapeutic diets for type 2 diabetes. J Nutr. 2011;141(8):1469-74.

320. Knowler WC, Barrett-Connor E, et al. Reduction in the incidence of type 2 diabetes with lifestyle intervention or metformin. *N Engl J Med.* 2002;346(6):393-403. http://www.ncbi.nlm.nih.gov.

321. Orchard TJ, Temprosa M, Goldberg R, et al. The effect of metformin and intensive lifestyle intervention on the metabolic syndrome: the Diabetes Prevention Program randomized trial. *Ann Intern Med.* 2005;142(8):611-9. http://www.ncbi.nlm.nih.gov.

322. Schulze MB, Hu FB. Primary prevention of diabetes: what can be done and how much can be prevented? Annu Rev Public Health. 2005;26:445-67. http://www.ncbi.nlm.nih.gov.

323. Wang Y, Rimm EB, Stampfer MJ, Willett WC, Hu FB. Comparison of abdominal adiposity and overall obesity in predicting risk of type 2 diabetes among men. Am J Clin Nutr. 2005;81(3):555-63.

324. Fox KA. Despres JP, Richard AJ, et al. Does abdominal obesity have a similar impact on cardiovascular disease and diabetes? A study of 91,246 ambulant patients in 27 European countries. Eur Heart J. 2009;30(24):3055-63. http://www.ncbi.nlm.nih.gov.

325. Huxley R, James WP, Barzi F, et al. Ethnic comparisons of the cross-sectional relationships between measures of body size with diabetes and hypertension. Obes Rev. 2008;9 Suppl 1:53-61. http://www.ncbi.nlm.nih.gov.

326. Bergstrom RW, Newell-Morris LL, Leonetti DL, et al. Association of elevated C-peptide level and increased intra-abdominal fat distribution with development of NIDDM in Japanese-American men. Bergstrom R. Diabetes. 1990;39(1):104-11. http://www.ncbi.nlm.nih.gov.

327. Deurenberg P, Deurenbery-Yap M,Guricci S. Asians are different from Caucasians and from each other in their body mass index/body fat per cent relationship. Obes Rev. 2002;3(3):141-6. http://www.ncbi.nlm.nih.gov.

328. Deurenberg P, Yap M, van Staveren WA. Body mass index and percent body fat: a meta analysis among different ethnic groups.Int J Obes Relat Metab Disord. 1998;22(12):1164-71. http://www.ncbi.nlm.nih.gov.

329. Lear SA, Humphries KH, Kohli S, et al. Visceral adipose tissue accumulation differs according to ethnic background: results of the Multicultural Community Health Assessment Trial (M-CHAT). Am J Clin Nutr. 2007;86(2):353-9. http://www.ncbi.nlm.nih.gov.

330. Hu F. Globalization of diabetes: the role of diet, lifestyle, and genes. Diabetes Care. 2011;34(6):1249-57. http://www.ncbi.nlm.nih.gov.

331. Qi L, Cornelis MC, Zhang C, van Dam RM, Hu FB. Genetic predisposition, Genetic Predisposition,Western dietary pattern, and the risk of type 2 diabetes in men. Am J Clin Nutr. 2009;89(5):1453-8. http://www.ncbi.nlm.nih.gov.

332. Cândido FG, Silva Ton WT, Gonçalves Alfenas Rde C. Dairy products consumption versus type 2 diabetes prevention and treatment; a review of recent findings from human studies. *Nutr Hosp.* 2013;28(5):1384-95. http://www.ncbi.nlm.nih.gov.

333. Gao D. et al. Dairy products consumption and risk of type 2 diabetes: systematic review and dose-response meta-analysis. *PLoS One.* 2013;8(9):e73965. http://www.ncbi.nlm.nih.gov.

334. Aune D. Dairy products and the risk of type 2 diabetes: a systematic review and dose-response meta-analysis of cohort studies. *Am J Clin Nutr.* 2013;98(4):1066-83. http://www.ncbi.nlm.nih.gov.

335. Pan A, Sun Q, Bernstein AM, Schulze MB, Manson JE, Willett WC, Hu FB. Red meat consumption and risk of type 2 diabetes: 3 cohorts of US adults and an updated meta-analysis. *Am J Clin Nutr.* 2011;94(4):1088-96. http://www.ncbi.nlm.nih.gov.

336. Fung TT, Schulze M, Manson JE, Willett WC, Hu FB. Dietary patterns, meat intake, and the risk of type 2 diabetes in women. *Arch Intern Med.* 2004;164(20):2235-40. http://www.ncbi.nlm.nih.gov.

337. Aune D, Ursin G, Veierød MB. Meat consumption and the risk of type 2 diabetes: a systematic review and meta-analysis of cohort studies. *Diabetologia.* 2009;52(11):2277-87. http://www.ncbi.nlm.nih.gov.

338. Esposito K, Kastorini CM, Panagiotakos DB, Giugliano D. Prevention of type 2 diabetes by dietary patterns: a systematic review of prospective studies and meta-analysis. *Metab Syndr Relat Disord.* 2010;8(6):471-6. http://www.ncbi.nlm.nih.gov.

339. van Dam RM, Willett WC, Rimm EB, Stampfer MJHu FB . Dietary patterns and risk for type 2 diabetes mellitus in U.S. men. *Ann Intern Med.* 2002;136(3):201-9. http://www.ncbi.nlm.nih.gov.

340. Song Y, Manson JE, Buring JE, Liu S. A prospective study of red meat consumption and type 2 diabetes in middle-aged and elderly women: the women's health study. *Diabetes Care.* 2004;27(9):2108:15. http://www.ncbi.nlm.nih.gov.

341. Barnard N, Levin S, Trapp C. Meat consumption as a risk factor for type 2 diabetes. Nutrients. 2014;6:897-910. http://www.ncbi.nlm.nih.gov.

342. Rajpathak S, Ma J, Manson J, Willett WC, Hu FB. Iron intake and the risk of type 2 diabetes in women: a prospective cohort study. *Diabetes Care.* 2006;29(6):1370-6. http://www.ncbi.nlm.nih.gov.

343. Lee DH, Folsom AR, Jacobs DR Jr. Dietary iron intake and Type 2 diabetes incidence in postmenopausal women: the Iowa Women's Health Study. Diabetologia. 2004;47(2):185-94. http://www.ncbi.nlm.nih.gov.

344. Jiang R, Ma J, Ascherio A, Stampfer MJ, Willett WC, Hu FB.Dietary iron intake and blood donations in relation to risk of type 2 diabetes in men: a prospective cohort study. Am J Clin Nutr. 2004;79(1):70-5. http://www.ncbi.nlm.nih.gov.

345. Bowers K, Yeung E, Williams MA, Qi L, Tobias DK, Hu FB, Zhang C. A Prospective Study of Prepregnancy Dietary Iron Intake and Risk for Gestational Diabetes Mellitus. *Diabetes Care.* 2011;34(7):1557-63. http://www.ncbi.nlm.nih.gov.

346. Qiu C, Zhang C, Gelaye B, Enquobahrie DA, Frederick IO, Williams MA. Gestational diabetes mellitus in relation to maternal dietary heme iron and nonheme iron intake. *Diabetes Care.* 2011;34(7):1564-9. http://www.ncbi.nlm.nih.gov.

347. Bowers K, Tobias DK, Yeung E, Hu FB, Zhang C. A prospective study of prepregnancy dietary fat intake and risk of gestational diabetes. *Am J Clin Nutr.* 2012;95(2):446-53.

348. Song Y, Manson JE, Buring JE, Sesso HD, Liu S. Associations of dietary flavonoids with risk of type 2 diabetes, and markers of insulin resistance and systemic inflammation in women: a prospective study and cross-sectional analysis. *J Am Coll Nutr.* 2005;24(5):376-84. http://www.ncbi.nlm.nih.gov.

349. Rizzo NS, Sabaté J, Jaceldo-Siegl K, Fraser GE. Vegetarian Dietary Patterns Are Associated With a Lower Risk of Metabolic Syndrome. *Diabetes Care.* 2011;34(5): 1225–1227. http://www.ncbi.nlm.nih.gov.

350. Wedick NM, Pan A, Cassidy A, Rimm EB, Sampson L, Rosner B, Willett W, Hu FB, Sun Q, van Dam RM. Dietary flavonoid intakes and risk of type 2 diabetes in US men and women. *Am J Clin Nutr. 2012;95(4):925-33.* http://www.ncbi.nlm.nih.gov.

351. Knekt P, Kumpulainen J, Järvinen R, et al. Flavonoid intake and risk of chronic diseases. *Am J Clin Nutr.* 2002;76(3):560-8. http://www.ncbi.nlm.nih.gov.

352. Janssens JP, et al. Molenberghs G. Effects of soft drink and table beer consumption on insulin response in normal teenagers and carbohydrate drink in youngsters. *Eur J Cancer Prev.* 1999;8:289–295. http://www.ncbi.nlm.nih.gov.

353. Bleich SN, Wang YC. Consumption of sugar-sweetened beverages among adults with type 2 diabetes. *Diabetes Care.* 2011;34(3):551-5. http://www.ncbi.nlm.nih.gov.

354. Odegaard AO, Koh WP, Arakawa K, Yu MC, Pereira MA. Soft drink and juice

consumption and risk of physician-diagnosed incident type 2 diabetes: the Singapore Chinese Health Study. *Am J Epidemiol.* 2010;171(6):701-8. http://www.ncbi.nlm.nih.gov.

355. Malik VS, Popkin BM, Bray GA, Després JP, Willett WC, Hu FB. Sugar-sweetened beverages and risk of metabolic syndrome and type 2 diabetes: a meta-analysis. *Diabetes Care.* 2010;33(11):2477-83. http://www.ncbi.nlm.nih.gov.

356. Dong JY, Xun P, He K, Qin LQ. Magnesium intake and risk of type 2 diabetes: meta-analysis of prospective cohort studies. *Diabetes Care.* 2011;34(9):2116-22. http://www.ncbi.nlm.nih.gov.

357. Chaudhary DP, Sharma R, Bansal DD. Implications of magnesium deficiency in type 2 diabetes: a review. *Biol Trace Elem Res.* 2010;134(2):119-29. http://www.ncbi.nlm.nih.gov.

358. van Dam RM, Hu FB, Rosenberg L, Krishnan S, Palmer JR. Dietary calcium and magnesium, major food sources, and risk of type 2 diabetes in U.S. black women. *Diabetes Care.* 2006;29(10):2238-43. http://www.ncbi.nlm.nih.gov.

359. Shaikh S, Karira KA. Magnesium deficiency in heart failure patients with diabetes mellitus. *J Pak Med Assoc.* 2011;61(9):901-3. http://www.ncbi.nlm.nih.gov.

360. Larsson SC, Wolk A. Magnesium intake and risk of type 2 diabetes: a meta-analysis. *J Intern Med.* 2007;262(2):208-14. http://www.ncbi.nlm.nih.gov.

361. Schulze MB, Schulz M, Heidemann C, Schienkiewitz A, Hoffmann K, Boeing H. Fiber and magnesium intake and incidence of type 2 diabetes: a prospective study and meta-analysis. *Arch Intern Med.* 2007;167(9):956-65. http://www.ncbi.nlm.nih.gov.

362. Jiang R, Manson JE, Stampfer MJ, Liu S, Willett WC, Hu FB. Nut and peanut butter consumption and risk of type 2 diabetes in women. *JAMA.* 2002;288(20):2554-60. http://www.ncbi.nlm.nih.gov.

363. Joergensen C, Reinhard H, Schmedes A, et al. Vitamin D levels and asymptomatic coronary artery disease in type 2 diabetic patients with elevated urinary albumin excretion rate. *Diabetes Care.* 2012;35(1):168-72. http://www.ncbi.nlm.nih.gov.

364. Joergensen C, Gall MA, Schmedes A, Tarnow L, Parving HH, Rossing P. Vitamin D levels and mortality in type 2 diabetes. *Diabetes Care.* 2010;33(10):2238-43. http://www.ncbi.nlm.nih.gov.

365. Gupta AK, Brashear MM, Johnson WD. Prediabetes and Prehypertension in Healthy Adults Are Associated With Low Vitamin D Levels. *Diabetes Care. 2011*; 34(3): 658–660.

366. Gupta AK, Brashear MM, Johnson WD. Low vitamin D levels, prediabetes and prehypertension in healthy African American adults. *Nutr Metab Cardiovasc*

Dis. 2012;22(10):877-82. http://www.ncbi.nlm.nih.gov.

367. Barengolts E. Vitamin D role and use in prediabetes. *Endocr Pract.* 2010;16(3):476-85. http://www.ncbi.nlm.nih.gov.

368. Pittas AG, Nelson J, Mitri J, et al. Plasma 25-hydroxyvitamin D and progression to diabetes in patients at risk for diabetes: an ancillary analysis in the Diabetes Prevention Program. *Diabetes Care.* 2012; 35(3): 565-573 . http://www.ncbi.nlm.nih.gov.

369. Gill JM, Cooper AR. Physical activity and prevention of type 2 diabetes mellitus. *Sports Med.* 2008;38(10):807-24. http://www.ncbi.nlm.nih.gov.

370. Hu G, Lindström J, Valle TT, Eriksson JG, Jousilahti P, Silventoinen K, Qiao Q, Tuomilehto J. Physical activity, body mass index, and risk of type 2 diabetes in patients with normal or impaired glucose regulation. *Arch Intern Med.* 2004;164(8):892-6. http://www.ncbi.nlm.nih.gov.

371. Hu G, Rico-Sanz J, Lakka TA, Tuomilehto J. Exercise, genetics and prevention of type 2 diabetes. *Essays Biochem.* 2006;42:177-92. http://www.ncbi.nlm.nih.gov.

372. Hu G, Lakka TA, Kilpeläinen TO, Tuomilehto J. Epidemiological studies of exercise in diabetes prevention. *Appl Physiol Nutr Metab.* 2007;32(3):583-95. http://www.ncbi.nlm.nih.gov.

373. Umpierre D, Ribeiro PA, Kramer CK, Leitão CB, Zucatti AT, Azevedo MJ, Gross JL, Ribeiro JP, Schaan BD. Physical activity advice only or structured exercise training and association with HbA1c levels in type 2 diabetes: a systematic review and meta-analysis. *JAMA.*2011;305(17):1790-9. http://www.ncbi.nlm.nih.gov.

374. Church TS, Blair SN, Cocreham S, et al. Effects of aerobic and resistance training on hemoglobin A1c levels in patients with type 2 diabetes: a randomized controlled trial. *JAMA.* 2010;304(20):2253-62. http://www.ncbi.nlm.nih.gov.

375. Sigal RJ, Kenny GP, Boulé NG, et al. Effects of aerobic training, resistance training, or both on glycemic control in type 2 diabetes: a randomized trial. *Ann Intern Med.* 2007;147(6):357-69. http://www.ncbi.nlm.nih.gov.

376. Misra A, Alappan NK, Vikram NK, Goel K, Gupta N, Mittal K, Bhatt S, Luthra K. Effect of supervised progressive resistance-exercise training protocol on insulin sensitivity, glycemia, lipids, and body composition in Asian Indians with type 2 diabetes. *Diabetes Care.* 2008;31(7):1282-7. http://www.ncbi.nlm.nih.gov.

377. Chudyk A, Petrella RJ. Effects of exercise on cardiovascular risk factors in type 2 diabetes: a meta-analysis. *Diabetes Care.* 2011;34(5):1228-37. http://www.ncbi.nlm.nih.gov.

378. Hu FB, Li TY, Colditz GA, Willett WC, Manson JE. Television Watching and Other Sedentary Behaviors in Relation to Risk of Obesity and Type 2 Diabetes Mellitus in Women. JAMA. 2003;289(14):1785-91.

379. Hegde SV, Adhikari P, Kotian S, Pinto VJ, D'Souza S, D'Souza V. Effect of 3-month yoga on oxidative stress in type 2 diabetes with or without complications: a controlled clinical trial. *Diabetes Care.* 2011;34(10):2208-10. http://www.ncbi.nlm.nih.gov.

380. Yang K, Bernardo LM, Sereika SM, Conroy MB, Balk J, Burke LE. Utilization of 3-month yoga program for adults at high risk for type 2 diabetes: a pilot study. *Evid Based Complement Alternat Med.* 2011;2011:257891. http://www.ncbi.nlm.nih.gov.

381. Zhang L, Curhan GC, Hu FB, et al. Association Between Passive and Active Smoking and Incident Type 2 Diabetes in Women. *Diabetes Care.* 20111; 34(4): 892–897. http://www.ncbi.nlm.nih.gov.

382. Xie X, Liu Q, Wu J, Wakui M. Impact of cigarette smoking in type 2 diabetes development. Acta Pharmacologica Sinica.2009;30:784–787.

383. National Diabetes Fact Sheet:National Diabetes Fact Sheet: Diagnosed and undiagnosed diabetes in the United States, all ages, 2010. Atlanta, GA: Centers for Disease and Control; 2011.

384. Xiang AH, Li BH, Black MH, et al. Racial and ethnic disparities in diabetes risk after gestational diabetes mellitus. *Diabetologia. 2011;54(12):3016-21.* http://www.ncbi.nlm.nih.gov.

385. Krishnan S, Rosenberg L, Djoussé L, Cupples LA, Palmer JR. Overall and central obesity and risk of type 2 diabetes in U.S. black women. *Obesity (Silver Spring).* 2007;15(7):1860-6. http://www.ncbi.nlm.nih.gov.

386. Tobias DK, Zhang C, van Dam RM, Bowers K, Hu FB. Physical activity before and during pregnancy and risk of gestational diabetes mellitus: a meta-analysis. *Diabetes Care.* 2011;34(1):223-9. http://www.ncbi.nlm.nih.gov.

387. Harizopoulou VC, et al. Maternal physical activity before and during early pregnancy as a risk factor for gestational diabetes mellitus. *Acta Diabetol.* 2010;47 Suppl 1:83-9. http://www.ncbi.nlm.nih.gov.

388. Dempsey JC, Sorensen TK, Williams MA, Lee IM, Miller RS, Dashow EE, Luthy DA. Prospective study of gestational diabetes mellitus risk in relation to maternal recreational physical activity before and during pregnancy. *Am J Epidemiol.* 2004 1;159(7):663-70. http://www.ncbi.nlm.nih.gov.

389. O'Reilly M, Avalos G, Dennedy MC, O'Sullivan EP, Dunne FP. Breast-feeding is associated with reduced postpartum maternal glucose intolerance after gestational diabetes. *Ir Med J. 2012;105(5 Suppl):31-6.* http://www.ncbi.nlm.nih.gov.

390. O'Reilly MW, Avalos G, Dennedy MC, O'Sullivan EP, Dunne F. Atlantic DIP: high prevalence of abnormal glucose tolerance post partum is reduced by breast-feeding in women with prior gestational diabetes mellitus. *Eur J Endocrinol.* 2011;165(6):953-9. http://www.ncbi.nlm.nih.gov.

391. Ziegler AG, Wallner M, Kaiser I, et al. Long-Term Protective Effect of Lactation on the Development of Type 2 Diabetes in Women With Recent Gestational Diabetes Mellitus. *Diabetes.* 2012;61(12):3167-71. http://www.ncbi.nlm.nih.gov.

392. Kjos SL, Henry O, Lee RM, Buchanan TA, Mishell DR Jr. The effect of lactation on glucose and lipid metabolism in women with recent gestational diabetes. *Obstet Gynecol.* 1993;82(3):451-5. http://www.ncbi.nlm.nih.gov.

393. Gunderson EP, Hedderson MM, Chiang V, et al. Lactation Intensity and Postpartum Maternal Glucose Tolerance and Insulin Resistance in Women With Recent GDM. *Diabetes Care.* 2012;35(1):50-56 . http://www.ncbi.nlm.nih.gov.

394. Top hypertension drugs in the United States based on revenue in 2011-2012 (in million U.S. dollars). Statista. http://www.statista.com.

395. Forman JP, Stampfer MJ, Curhan GC. Diet and lifestyle risk factors associated with incident hypertension in women. *JAMA.* 2009;302(4):401-11. http://www.ncbi.nlm.nih.gov.

396. Pettersen BJ, Anousheh R, Fan J, Jaceldo-Siegl K, Fraser GE. Vegetarian diets and blood pressure among white subjects: results from the Adventist Health Study-2 (AHS-2). *Public Health Nutr.* 2012; 15(10): 1909–1916. http://www.ncbi.nlm.nih.gov.

397. Berkow SE, Barnard ND. Blood pressure regulation and vegetarian diets. *Nutr Rev.* 2005;63(1):1-8. http://www.ncbi.nlm.nih.gov.

398. Rouse IL, Armstrong BK, Beilin LJ. The relationship of blood pressure to diet and lifestyle in two religious populations. *J Hypertens.* 1983;1(1):65-71. http://www.ncbi.nlm.nih.gov.

399. Kushi LH, Lenart EB, Willett WC. Plant foods and dairy products. *Am J Clin Nutr.* 1995; 61(suppl): 1407S-1415S. http://www.ncbi.nlm.nih.gov.

400. Langreth R. *Just Say No.* . Forbes Magazine; Nov 29, 2004.

401. Jenkins DJ, Kendall CW, Marchie A et al. Direct comparison of a dietary portfolio of cholesterol-lowering foods with a statin in hypercholesterolemic participants. *Am J Clin Nutr.* 2005 Feb;81(2):380-7.

402. Becker DJ, Gordon RY, Halbert SC, et al. Red yeast rice for dyslipidmia in statin-intolerant patients. *Annals of Internal Medicine.*2009;150(12):830-839. http://www.ncbi.nlm.nih.gov.

403. Racial/ethnic and socioeconomic disparities in multiple risk factors for heart disease and stroke – United States 2003. MMWR. Centers for Disease Control and Prevention.2005;54(05):113-117. http://www.cdc.gov.

404. Inpatient Surgery - Data are for the U.S. Hyattsville, MD: National Center for Health Statistics; 2010. http://www.cdc.gov/nchs/fastats/insurg.

405. Heart Disease Risk Factors. Atlanta, GA: Centers for Disease Control and Prevention; 2009. http://www.cdc.gov.

406. National Coverage Determination (NCD) for Intensive Cardiac Rehabilitation (ICR) Programs. Centers for Medicare and Medicaid Services. U.S. Department of Health and Human Services. http://www.cms.gov.

407. Ornish D, Brown SE, Scherwitz LW, Billings JH, Armstrong WT, Ports TA, McLanahan SM, Kirkeeide RL, Brand RJ, Gould KL. Can lifestyle changes reverse coronary heart disease? The Lifestyle Heart Trial. *Lancet.* 1990;336(8708):129-33. http://www.ncbi.nlm.nih.gov.

408. Ornish D, Scherwitz LW, Billings JH, et al. Intensive lifestyle changes for reversal of coronary heart disease. *JAMA.* 1998;280(23):2001-7. http://www.ncbi.nlm.nih.gov.

409. Pischke CR, Weidner G, Elliott-Eller M, Ornish D. Lifestyle changes and clinical profile in coronary heart disease patients with an ejection fraction of <or=40% or >40% in the Multicenter Lifestyle Demonstration Project. *Eur J Heart Fail.* 2007;9(9):928-34. http://www.ncbi.nlm.nih.gov.

410. Pischke CR, Elliott-Eller M, Li M, Mendell N, Ornish D, Weidner G. Clinical events in coronary heart disease patients with an ejection fraction of 40% or less: 3-year follow-up results. *J Cardiovasc Nurs.* 2010;25(5):E8-E15. http://www.ncbi.nlm.nih.gov.

411. Capewell S, O'Flaherty M. Can dietary changes rapidly decrease cardiovascular mortality rates? *Eur Heart J.*2011; 32 (10):1187-1189. http://www.ncbi.nlm.nih.gov.

412. U.S. Cancer Statistics Working Group. United States Cancer Statistics: 1999–2009 Incidence and Mortality Web-based Report. Atlanta, Ga: U.S. Department of Health and Human Services, Centers for Disease Control and and National Cancer Institute; 2013. http://www.cdc.gov/uscs. Prevention.

413. Kritz FL Cancer patients facing costly treatment can benefit from frank talks with doctors. Los Angeles, CA: LA Times. Feb 16, 2009. http:// www.articles.latimes.com.

414. Kolata G, Pollack A. Costly cancer drug offers hope, but also a dilemma. New York Times. Jul 6, 2008. http://www.nytimes.com.

415. Bach PB, Saltz LB, Wittes RE. In cancer care, cost matters. New York Times. Oct 14, 2012. http://www.nytimes.com.

416. Ramsey SD, Fedorenko CR, Snell KS, et al. Cancer diagnosis as a risk factor for personal bankruptcy. *J Clin Oncol 29:* 2011 (suppl; abstr 6007). http://www.ncbi.nlm.nih.gov.

417. The 2006 Cancer Fact Book. Bethesda, MD: National Institutes of Health/US Health and Human Services; 2006. http://obf.cancer.gov.

418. National Cancer Institute FY 2011 Budget. Bethesda, MD: National Cancer Institute/Health and Human Services; 2011.http://officeofbudget.od.nih.gov

419. National Cancer Institute FY Budget 2014. Bethesda, MD: National Cancer Institute/US Health and Human Services;2014.http://obf.cancer.gov.

420. FY 2005 - FY 2014 cancer prevention and control program funding. Atlanta, GA: Centers for Disease Control and Prevention;2014.

421. FY 2005 - FY 2014 funding - national comprehensive cancer control program. Atlanta, Georgia: Centers for Disease Control and Prevention;2014.

422. McMillen R, Hill A, Valentine N, Collins R. The Starkville & Hattiesburg Heart Attack Studies. Starksville, MS: Mississippi State University Social Science Research Center;2010. http: www.ttac.org.

423. State Cancer Profiles. Bethesda, MD: US Department of Health and Human Services. 2013. http://www.statecancerprofiles.cancer.gov.

424. 100% smoke-free communities in Mississippi. Mississippi Tobacco Data. Starksville, MS: Social Science Research Center. Mississippi State University; 2014. http://www.http://surveillance.mstobaccodata.org.

425. American Lung Association. State of Tobacco Control 2013. Washington, DC: American Lung Association; 2013. http:// www.stateoftobaccocontrol.org.

426. Overview of the Family Smoking Prevention and Tobacco Control Act. Rockville, MD: Center for Tobacco Products. http://www.fda.gov/downloads/TobaccoProducts/GuidanceComplianceRegulatoryInformation/UCM237080.pdf.

427. Levy DT, Pearson JL, Villanti AC, et al. Modeling the Future Effects of a Menthol Ban on Smoking Prevalence and Smoking-Attributable Deaths in the United States. *Am J Public Health*. 2011;101(7):1236-40. http://www.ncbi.nlm.nih.gov.

428. The FDA Center for Tobacco Products. FDA Remarks on the Report and Recommendation on the Public Health Impact of Menthol Cigarettes. Silverspring, MD: USFDA;2011. http://www.fda.gov.

429. Tobacco Products Scientific Advisory Committee. Menthol Cigarettes and Public Health: Review of the Scientific Evidence and Recommendations. Silverspring, MD: USFDA; 2011. http://www.fda.gov.

430. Deyton LR. FDA Remarks on the Report and Recommendation on the Public Health Impact of Menthol Cigarettes. Silver Springs, MD: US Food and Drug Administration; 2011. http://www.fda.gov.

431. Preliminary scientific evaluation of the possible health effects of menthol versus nonmenthol cigarettes. Silver Spring, MD: USFDA; 2013. http://www.fda.gov.

432. Menthol in Cigarettes, Tobacco Products; Request for Comments. 21 CFR Part 1140. Silver Spring, MD: USFDA;2013. http://www.gpo.gov/fdsys/pkg/FR-2013-07-24/pdf/2013-17805.pdf.

433. FDA takes step to further reduce trans fats in processed foods. Silver Spring, MD:Food and Drug Administration; 2013. http://www.fda.gov.

434. Master Settlement Agreement. http://publichealthlawcenter.org/sites/default/files/resources/master-settlement-agreement.pdf;1998.

435. Broken Promises to Our Children - The 1998 State Tobacco Settlement 15 Years Later. Washington, DC: Campaign for Tobacco Free Kids. http://www.tobaccofreekids.org/content/what_we_do/state_local_issues/settlement/FY2014/StateSettlementReport_FY2014.pdf;2013.

436. Ramirez A. A Cigarette Campaign Under Fire. New York, NY: New York Times. Jan 12, 1990. http://www.nytimes.com.

437. Rising J, Alexander L. Marketing of menthol cigarettes and consumer perceptions. *Tob Induc Dis.* 2011;9 Suppl 1:S2. http://www.ncbi.nlm.nih.gov.

438. Landrine H, Klonoff EA, Fernandez S, et al. Cigarette advertising in Black, Latino, and White magazines, 1998-2002: an exploratory investigation. *Ethn Dis.* 2005 Winter;15(1):63-7. http://www.ncbi.nlm.nih.gov.

439. Tobacco - Lobbying. Washington, DC:Center for Responsive Politics; 2013. http://www.opensecrets.org.

440. Andreaff M, Goodrich D, Pardee AB. Chapter 2 Cell Proliferation, Differentiation, and Apoptosis. In: Bast RcC Kufe DW, Pollock RE et al. Holland-Frei Cancer Medicine 5th edition. Hamilton (ON):

441. Harms of Smoking and Health Benefits of Quitting. Bethesda, MD: National Cancer Institute; 2013. http://www.cancer.gov.

442. Harms of Smoking and Health Benefits of Quitting. Bethesda, MD: National Cancer Institute; 2013. http://www.cancer.gov.

443. When smokers quit — what are the benefits over time? Atlanta, GA: American Cancer Soceity; 2012. http://www.cancer.org.

444. Ogden GR. Alcohol and oral cancer. *Alcohol.* 2005;35(3):169-73. http://www.ncbi.nlm.nih.gov.

445. Ide R, Mizoue T, Fujino Y, et al. Cigarette smoking, alcohol drinking, and oral and pharyngeal cancer mortality in Japan. *Oral Dis.* 2008;14(4):314-9. http://www.ncbi.nlm.nih.gov.

446. IARC Monographs on the evaluation of carcinogenic risks to humans. Vol 44. Alcohol drinking. France: International Agency for Research on Cancer; 1988. http://www.monographs.iarc.

447. Cho E, Lee JE, Rimm EB, et al. Alcohol consumption and the risk of colon cancer by family history of colorectal cancer1. *Am J Clin Nutr.* 2012; 95(2):413–419. http://www.ncbi.nlm.nih.gov.

448. Alcohol Use and Cancer. The American Cancer Society. Atlanta, GA. http://www.cancer.org.

449. Li CI, Chlebowski RT, Freiberg M, et al. Alcohol Consumption and Risk of Postmenopausal Breast Cancer by Subtype: The Women's Health Initiative Observational Study. *J Natl Cancer Inst.* 2010; 102(18): 1422–1431. http://www.ncbi.nlm.nih.gov.

450. Kabat GC, Kim M, Phipps AI, et al. Smoking and alcohol consumption in relation to risk of triple-negative breast cancer in a cohort of postmenopausal women. *Cancer Causes Control.* 2011; 22(5) 775–783. http://www.ncbi.nlm.nih.gov.

451. Singletary KW, Gapstur SM. Alcohol and breast cancer: review of epidemiologic and experimental evidence and potential mechanisms. *JAMA.* 2001;286:2143–51. http://www.ncbi.nlm.nih.gov.

452. Dumitrescu RG, Shields PG. The etiology of alcohol-induced breast cancer. *Alcohol.* 2005;35:213–25. http://www.ncbi.nlm.nih.gov.

453. Maskarinec G, Morimoto Y, Takata Y, et al. Alcohol and dietary fibre intakes affect circulating sex hormones among premenopausal women. *Public Health Nutr.* 2006;9:875–81. http://www.ncbi.nlm.nih.gov.

454. Hong J, Holcomb VB, Dang F, Porampornpilas K, Núñez NP. Alcohol Consumption, Obesity, Estrogen Treatment and Breast Cancer. *Anticancer Res.* 2010;30(1):1-8. http://www.ncbi.nlm.nih.gov.

455. Kwan ML, Kushi LH, Weltzien E, et. al. Alcohol Consumption and Breast Cancer Recurrence and Survival Among Women With Early-Stage Breast Cancer: The Life After Cancer Epidemiology Study. *J Clin Oncol.* 2010; 28(29):4410–4416. http://www.ncbi.nlm.nih.gov.

456. Li CI, Daling JR, Porter PL, Tang MT, Malone KE. Relationship between potentially modifiable lifestyle factors and risk of second primary contralateral breast cancer among women diagnosed with estrogen receptor-positive invasive breast cancer. *J Clin Oncol.* 2009;27(32):5312-8. http://www.ncbi.nlm.nih.gov.

457. Sellers TA, Vierkant RA, Cerhan JR, et al. Interaction of dietary folate intake, alcohol, and risk of hormone receptor-defined breast cancer in a prospective study of postmenopausal women. *Cancer Epidemiol Biomarkers Prev.* 2002;11(10 Pt 1):1104-7. http://www.ncbi.nlm.nih.gov.

458. Sellers TA, Kushi LH, Cerhan JR, et. al. Dietary folate intake, alcohol, and risk of breast cancer in a prospective study of postmenopausal women. Epidemiology. 2001;12(4):420-8. http://www.ncbi.nlm.nih.gov.

459. Baglietto L, English DR, Gertig DM, et.al. Does dietary folate intake modify effect of alcohol consumption on breast cancer risk? Prospective cohort study. *BMJ*. 2005; 331(7520): 807. http://www.ncbi.nlm.nih.gov.

460. Zhang SM, Hankinson SE, Hunter DJ, Giovannucci EL, Colditz GA, Willett WC. Folate intake and risk of breast cancer characterized by hormone receptor status. *Cancer Epidemiol Biomarkers Prev*. 2005;14(8):2004-8. http://www.ncbi.nlm.nih.gov.

461. Zhang S, Hunter DJ, Hankinson SE, Giovannucci EL, Rosner BA, Colditz GA, Speizer FE, Willett WC. A prospective study of folate intake and the risk of breast cancer. *JAMA*. 1999;281(17):1632-7. http://www.ncbi.nlm.nih.gov.

462. Renehan AG, Tyson M, Egger M. Body-mass index and incidence of cancer: a systematic review and meta-analysis of prospective observational studies. *The Lancet*.2008;371(9612):569–578. http://www.ncbi.nlm.nih.gov.

463. Li D, Morris JS, Liu J, Hassan MM, Day RS, Bondy ML, Abbruzzese JL. Body mass index and risk, age of onset, and survival in patients with pancreatic cancer. *JAMA*. 2009;301(24):2553-62. http://www.ncbi.nlm.nih.gov.

464. Grönberg H, Damber L, Damber JE. Total food consumption and body mass index in relation to prostate cancer risk: a case-control study in Sweden with prospectively collected exposure data. *Journal of Urology*. 1996;155(3):969–974. http://www.ncbi.nlm.nih.gov.

465. Snowdon DA, Phillips RL, Choi W. Body size and prostate cancer: a 20-year follow-up study among 135006 Swedish construction workers. *American Journal of Epidemiology*. 1984;120(2):244–250. http://www.ncbi.nlm.nih.gov.

466. Snowdon DA, Phillips RL, Choi W.Diet, obesity, and risk of fatal prostate cancer. *American Journal of Epidemiology*. 1984;120(2):244–250. http://www.ncbi.nlm.nih.gov.

467. Freedland SJ, Terris MK, Platz EA, Presti JC Jr. Body mass index as a predictor of prostate cancer: development versus detection on biopsy. *Urology*. 2005;66(1):108-13. http://www.ncbi.nlm.nih.gov.

468. Joshu CE, Mondul AM, Menke A, et al. Weight gain is associated with an increased risk of prostate cancer recurrence after prostatectomy in the PSA era. *Cancer Prev Res (Phila)*. 2011;4(4):544-51. http://www.ncbi.nlm.nih.gov.

469. Wu C, Aronson WJ, Terris MK, et al. Diabetes predicts metastasis after radical prostatectomy in obese men: results from the SEARCH database. *BJU Int. 2013*;111(8):E310-8. http://www.ncbi.nlm.nih.gov.

470. Freedland SJ, Bañez LL, Sun LL, Fitzsimons NJ, Moul JW. Obese men have higher-grade and larger tumors: an analysis of the duke prostate center database. *Prostate Cancer Prostatic Dis*. 2009;12(3):259-63. http://www.ncbi.nlm.nih.gov.

471. *Tumor Grade*. Bethesda, MD: National Institutes of Health; 2012. http://www.cancer.gov.

472. Calle EE, Rodriguez C, Walker-Thurmond K, Thun MJ. Overweight, obesity, and mortality from cancer in a prospectively studied cohort of U.S. adults. *N Engl J Med*. 2003;348(17):1625-38. http://www.ncbi.nlm.nih.gov.

473. Garfinkle, L. Overweight and Cancer. *Ann Intern Med*. 1985;103(6):1034-6. http://www.ncbi.nlm.nih.gov.

474. Møller H, Mellemgaard A, Lindvig K, Olsen JH. Obesity and cancer risk: a Danish record-linkage study. *Eur J Cancer*. 1994;30A(3):344-50. http://www.ncbi.nlm.nih.gov.

475. Harris HR, Willett WC, Terry KL, Michels KB. Body fat distribution and risk of premenopausal breast cancer in the Nurses' Health Study II. *J Natl Cancer Inst*. 2011;103(3):273-8. http://www.ncbi.nlm.nih.gov.

476. Harris HR, Willett WC, Terry KL, Michels KB. Body fat distribution and risk of premenopausal breast cancer in the Nurses' Health Study II. *J Natl Cancer Inst*. 2011;103(3):273-8. http://www.ncbi.nlm.nih.gov.

477. Triple Negative Breast Cancer. Bethesda, MD: National Cancer Institute. 2013. http://www.cancer.gov.

478. Davis AA, Kaklamani VG. Metabolic syndrome and triple-negative breast cancer. a new paradigm. *Int J Breast Cancer*. 2012;2012:809291. http://www.ncbi.nlm.nih.gov.

479. Anders C, Carey LA. Understanding and treating triple-negative breast cancer. *Oncology (Williston Park)*. 2008;22(11):1233-9. http://www.ncbi.nlm.nih.gov.

480. Carey L, Winer E, Viale G, Cameron D, Gianni L. Triple-negative breast cancer: disease entity or title of convenience? *Nature Reviews Clinical Oncology*. 2010;7(12):683–692. http://www.ncbi.nlm.nih.gov.

481. Eldridge L. What is the p53 Gene? http://www.lungcancer.about.com.

482. Lund MJ, Trivers KF, Porter PL, et al. Race and triple negative threats to breast cancer survival: a population-based study in Atlanta, GA. *Breast Cancer Res Treat*. 2009;113(2):357-70. http://www.ncbi.nlm.nih.gov.

483. Morris GJ, Naidu S, Topham AK, et al. Differences in breast carcinoma characteristics in newly diagnosed African-American and Caucasian patients: a single-institution compilation compared with the National Cancer Institute's Surveillance, Epidemiology, and End Results database. *Cancer*. 2007;110(4):876-84. http://www.ncbi.nlm.nih.gov.

484. Jones BA, Kasi SV, Curnen MG, Owens PH, Dubrow R. Severe obesity as an explanatory factor for the black/white difference in stage at diagnosis of breast cancer. *Am J Epidemiol*. 1997;146(5):394-404. http://www.ncbi.nlm.nih.gov.

485. Cui Y, Whiteman MK, Langenberg P, Sexton M, Tkaczuk KH, Flaws JA, Bush TL. Can obesity explain the racial difference in stage of breast cancer at diagnosis between black and white women? *J Womens Health Gend Based Med.* 2002;11(6):527-36. http://www.ncbi.nlm.nih.gov.

486. Connolly BS, Barnett C, Vogt KN, et al. A meta-analysis of published literature on waist-to-hip ratio and risk of breast cancer. *Nutrition and Cancer.*2002;44(2):127–138. http://www.ncbi.nlm.nih.gov.

487. Huang Z, Willett WC, Colditz GA, Hunter DJ, Manson JE, Rosner B, Speizer FE, Hankinson SE. Waist circumference, waist:hip ratio, and risk of breast cancer in the Nurses' Health Study. *Am J Epidemiol.* 1999;150(12):1316-24. http://www.ncbi.nlm.nih.gov.

488. Fagherazzi G, Chabbert-Buffet N, Fabre A, et al. Hip circumference is associated with the risk of premenopausal ER-/PR- breast cancer. *Int J Obes (Lond).* 2012;36(3):431-9. http://www.ncbi.nlm.nih.gov.

489. Giovannucci E, Ascherio A, Rimm EB, Colditz GA, Stampfer MJ, Willett WC. Physical activity, obesity, and risk for colon cancer and adenoma in men. *Ann Intern Med.* 1995;122(5):327-34. http://www.ncbi.nlm.nih.gov.

490. Zilli T, Nguyen TV, Bahary JP, et al. Prognostic impact of abdominal adiposity, waist circumference and body mass index in patients with intermediate-risk prostate cancer treated with radiotherapy. *Int J Obes (Lond).* 2011;35(11):1421-6. http://www.ncbi.nlm.nih.gov.

491. Nemesure B, Wu SY, Hennis A, et al. Central adiposity and Prostate Cancer in a Black Population. http://www.ncbi.nlm.nih.gov. *Cancer Epidemiol Biomarkers Prev.* 2012;21(5):851-8.

492. Blüher MK. The inflammatory process of adipose tissue. *Pediatr Endocrinol Rev.* 2008;6(1):24-31. http://www.ncbi.nlm.nih.gov.

493. Calle EE, Kaaks R. Overweight, obesity and cancer: epidemiological evidence and proposed. *Nature Reviews Cancer.* 2004;4(8):579–591. http://www.ncbi.nlm.nih.gov.

494. Schenk S, Saberi M, Olefsky JM. Insulin sensitivity: modulation by nutrients and inflammation. *Journal of Clinical Investigation.* 2008;118(9):2992–3002. http://www.ncbi.nlm.nih.gov.

495. de Luca C, Olefsky JM. Inflammation and insulin resistance. *FEBS Lett. 2008;582(1):97-105.* http://www.ncbi.nlm.nih.gov.

496. Ramos-Nino ME. The Role of Chronic Inflammation in Obesity-Associated Cancers. *ISRN Oncol.* 2013;2013:697521. http://www.ncbi.nlm.nih.gov.

497. Monteiro R, Azevedo I. Chronic inflammation in obesity and the metabolic syndrome. *Mediators Inflamm.* 2010;2010. pii: 289645. http://www.ncbi.nlm.nih.gov.

498. Vendramini-Costa DB, Carvalho JE. Molecular link mechanisms between inflammation and cancer. *Curr Pharm Des.* 2012;18(26):3831-52. http://www.ncbi.nlm.nih.gov.

499. Cohen SM, Purtilo DT, Ellwein LB. Ideas in pathology.Pivotal role of increased cell proliferation in human carcinogenesis. *Mod Pathol.* 1991;4: 371±82. http://www.ncbi.nlm.nih.gov.

500. Kuper H, Adami HO, Trichopoulos D. Infections as a major preventable cause of human cancer. *J Intern Med.* 2000;248(3):171-83. http://www.ncbi.nlm.nih.gov.

501. Kuper, H, Adami HO, Trichopoulos D. Infections as a major preventable cause of human cancer. *Journal of Internal Medicine* 2000; 248: 171±183. http://www.ncbi.nlm.nih.gov.

502. HPV and Cancer. Atlanta, GA. National Cancer Center Institute. National Institutes of Health. 2012. http:// cancer.gov/cancertopics/factsheet/Risk/HPV

503. Shoelson SE, Lee J, Goldfine AB. Inflammation and insulin resistance. *Journal of Clinical Investigation.* 2006;116(7):1793–1801. http://www.ncbi.nlm.nih.gov.

504. Kahn SE, Hull RL, Utzschneider KM. Mechanisms linking obesity to insulin resistance and type 2 diabetes. *Nature.* 2006;444(7121):840-6. http://www.ncbi.nlm.nih.gov.

505. Yu H, Rohan T. Role of the insulin-like growth factor family in cancer development and progression. *J Natl Cancer Inst.* 2000;92(18):1472-89. http://www.ncbi.nlm.nih.gov.

506. Renehan AG, Zwahlen M, Minder C, O'Dwyer ST, Shalet SM, Egger M. Insulin-like growth factor(IGF)-I, IGF binding protein-3, and cancer risk: systematic review and meta-regression analysis. *Lancet.* 2004;363(9418):1346–53. http://www.ncbi.nlm.nih.gov.

507. Calle EE, Kaaks R. Overweight, obesity and cancer: epidemiological evidence and proposed mechanisms. *Nat Rev Cancer.* 2004;4(8):579-91. http://www.ncbi.nlm.nih.gov.

508. Lawlor M A, Alessi D. PKB/Akt: a key mediator of cell proliferation, survival and insulin responses? *J Cell Sci.* 2001;114(Pt 16):2903-10. http://www.ncbi.nlm.nih.gov.

509. Khandwala H M, McCutcheon I E, Flyvbjerg A, Friend K E. The effects of insulin-like growth factors on tumorigenesis and neoplastic growth. *Endocr Rev.* 2000;21(3):215-44. http://www.ncbi.nlm.nih.gov.

510. Stattin P, Bylund A, Rinaldi S,. Plasma insulin-like growth factor-binding proteins, and prostate cancer risk: a prospective study. *J Natl Cancer Inst.* 2000;92(23):1910-7. http://www.ncbi.nlm.nih.gov.

511. Chan JM, et al. Plasma insulin-like growth factor-I and prostate cancer risk: a prospective study. *Science.* 1998;279(5350):563-6. http://www.ncbi.nlm.nih.gov.

512. Baglietto L, et al. Circulating concentrations of insulin-like growth factor-I and risk of breast cancer. *Cancer Epidemiol Biomarkers Prev.* 2007;16(4):763-8. http://www.ncbi.nlm.nih.gov.

513. Hankinson SE, et al. Circulating concentrations of insulin-like growth factor-I and risk of breast cancer. *Lancet.* 1998;351(9113):1393-6. http://www.ncbi.nlm.nih.gov.

514. Muti P, Quattrin T, Grant BJ,. Fasting glucose is a risk factor for breast cancer: a prospective study. *Cancer Epidemiol Biomarkers Prev.* 2002;11(11):1361-8. http://www.ncbi.nlm.nih.gov.

515. Kaaks R, Toniolo P, Akhmedkhanov A, et al. Serum C-peptide, insulin-like growth factor (IGF)-I, Igf-binding proteins, and colorectal cancer risk in women. *J Natl Cancer Inst.* 2000;92(19):1592-600. http://www.ncbi.nlm.nih.gov.

516. Schoen RE, Tangen CM, Kuller LH, et al. Increased blood glucose and insulin, body size, and incident colorectal cancer. *J Natl Cancer Inst.* 1999;91(13):1147-54. http://www.ncbi.nlm.nih.gov.

517. Cromie WJ. *Growth Factor Raises Cancer Risk.* Cambridge, MA: Harvard University;April 22, 1999. www.news.harvard.edu.

518. Moreira DM. The association of diabetes mellitus and high-grade prostate cancer in a multiethnic biopsy series. *Cancer Causes Control.* 2011Jul;22(7):977-83.

519. Wu C. et. al. Diabetes predicts metastasis after radical prostatectomy in obese men: results from the SEARCH database. *BJU Int.* 2013 June;111(8):E310-8.

520. Li C, Zhao G, Okoro CA, Wen XJ, Ford ES, Balluz LS. Prevalence of diagnosed cancer according to duration of diagnosed diabetes and current insulin use among U.S. Adults with diagnosed diabetes: findings from the 2009 behavioral risk factor surveillance system. *Diabetes Care.* 2013;36(6):1569-76. http://www.ncbi.nlm.nih.gov.

521. Hardefeldt PJ, Edirimanne S, Eslick GD. Diabetes increases the risk of breast cancer: a meta-analysis. *Endocr Relat Cancer.* 2012;19(6):793-803. http://www.ncbi.nlm.nih.gov.

522. Boyle P, Boniol M, Koechlin A, et al. Diabetes and breast cancer risk: a meta-analysis. *Br J Cancer.* 2012;107(9):1608-17. http://www.ncbi.nlm.nih.gov.

523. Bowker SL, Richardson K, Marra CA, Johnson JA. Risk of breast cancer after onset of type 2 diabetes: evidence of detection bias in postmenopausal women. *Diabetes Care.* 2011;34(12):2542-4. http://www.ncbi.nlm.nih.gov.

524. Ronco AL, De Stefani E, Deneo-Pellegrini H, Quarneti A. Diabetes, overweight and risk of postmenopausal breast cancer: a case-control study in Uruguay. *Asian Pac J Cancer Prev.* 2012;13(1):139-46. http://www.ncbi.nlm.nih.gov.

525. Liu X, Ji J, Sundquist K, Sundquist J, Hemminki K. The impact of type 2 diabetes mellitus on cancer-specific survival: a follow-up study in Sweden. *Cancer.* 2012;118(5):1353-61. http://www.ncbi.nlm.nih.gov.

526. Schrauder MG, Fasching PA, Häberle L, et al. Diabetes and prognosis in a breast cancer cohort. *J Cancer Res Clin Oncol.* 2011;137(6):975-83. http://www.ncbi.nlm.nih.gov.

527. Liu X, Ji J, Sundquist K, Sundquist J, Hemminki K. Mortality causes in cancer patients with type 2 diabetes mellitus. *Eur J Cancer Prev.* 2012;21(3):300-6. http://www.ncbi.nlm.nih.gov.

528. Li Z, Luo Y, Gong Y, Liu Y, Qiu W, Tu J. Clinical features and molecular phenotypes of breast cancer in patients with type-2 diabetes mellitus. *Asian Pac J Cancer Prev.* 2011;12(9):2183-8. http://www.ncbi.nlm.nih.gov.

529. Lipscombe LL, Goodwin PJ, Zinman B, McLaughlin JR, Hux JE. The impact of diabetes on survival following breast cancer. *Breast Cancer Res Treat.* 2008;109(2):389-95.

530. Erickson K, Patterson RE, Flatt SW, et al. Clinically defined type 2 diabetes mellitus and prognosis in early-stage breast cancer. *J Clin Oncol.* 2011;29(1):54-60.

531. Tammemagi CM, Nerenz D, Neslund-Dudas C, Feldkamp C, Nathanson D. Comorbidity and survival disparities among black and white patients with breast cancer. *JAMA.* 2005;294(14):1765-72. http://www.ncbi.nlm.nih.gov.

532. Braithwaite D, Tammemagi CM, Moore DH, et al. Hypertension is an independent predictor of survival disparity between African-American and white breast cancer patients. *Int J Cancer.* 2009;124(5):1213-9. http://www.ncbi.nlm.nih.gov.

533. Paxton RJ, Taylor WC, Chang S, Courneya KS, Jones LA. Lifestyle behaviors of african american breast cancer survivors: a sisters network, inc. Study. *PLoS One.* 2013;8(4):e61854. http://www.ncbi.nlm.nih.gov.

534. National Cancer Institute Dictionary. *Akt.* Bethesda, Md: National Cancer Institute. 2013. http://www.cancer.gov.

535. Lawlor MA, Alessi DR. PKB/Akt: a key mediator of cell proliferation, survival and insulin responses? *J Cell Sci.* 2001;114(Pt 16):2903-10. http://www.ncbi.nlm.nih.gov.

536. A Potential Sugar Fix for Tumors. Duke Medicine News and Communications. http:// www.dukehealth.org.

537. Li Y, Liang L, Tollefsbol TO. Glucose restriction can extend normal cell lifespan and impair precancerous cell growth through epigenetic control of hTERT and p16 expression. FASEB J. 2010; 24(5): 1442–1453.

http://www.ncbi.nlm.nih.gov.

538. Sieri S, Muti P, Claudia A, et al. Prospective study on the role of glucose metabolism in breast cancer occurrence. *Int J Cancer.* 2012;130(4):921-9. http://www.ncbi.nlm.nih.gov.

539. Contiero P, Berrino F, Tagliabue G, et al. Fasting blood glucose and long-term prognosis of non-metastatic breast cancer: a cohort study. *Breast Cancer Res Treat. 2013;* 138(3):951-9. http://www.ncbi.nlm.nih.gov.

540. Longo VD, Fontana L. Calorie restriction and cancer prevention: metabolic and molecular mechanisms. *Trends Pharmacol Sci.* 2010;31(2):89-98. http://www.ncbi.nlm.nih.gov.

541. Thissen JP, Ketelslegers JM, Underwood LE. Nutritional regulation of the insulin-like growth factors. *Endocr Rev.* 1994;15(1):80-101. http://www.ncbi.nlm.nih.gov.

542. Fontana L, Weiss EP, Villareal DT, Klein S, Holloszy JO. Long-term effects of calorie or protein restriction on serum IGF-1 and IGFBP-3 concentration in humans. *Aging Cell.* 2008;7(5):681-7. http://www.ncbi.nlm.nih.gov.

543. Giovannucci E, et. al. Nutritional predictors of insulin-like growth factor I and their relationships to cancer in men. *Cancer Epidemiol Biomarkers Prev.* 2003;12(2):84-9. http://www.ncbi.nlm.nih.gov.

544. Holmes MD, Pollak MN, Willett WC, Hankinson SE. Dietary correlates of plasma insulin-like growth factor I and insulin-like growth factor binding protein 3 concentrations. *Cancer Epidemiol Biomarkers Prev.* 2002;11(9):852-61. http://www.ncbi.nlm.nih.gov.

545. Philipps AF, Dvorák B, Kling PJ, Grille JG, Koldovský O. Absorption of milk-borne insulin-like growth factor-I into portal blood of suckling rats. *J Pediatr Gastroenterol Nutr.* 2000;31(2):128-35. http://www.ncbi.nlm.nih.gov.

546. Branch-Mays GL, Dawson DR, Gunsolley JC,. The effects of a calorie-reduced diet on periodontal inflammation and disease in a non-human primate model. *J Periodontol.* 2008;79(7):1184-91. http://www.ncbi.nlm.nih.gov.

547. Messaoudi I, Warner J, Fischer M, et al. Delay of T cell senescence by caloric restriction in aged long-lived nonhuman primates. *Proc Natl Acad Sci U S A. 2006;103(51):19448-53.* http://www.ncbi.nlm.nih.gov.

548. Colman RJ, et al. Caloric restriction delays disease onset and mortality in rhesus monkeys. *Science.* 2009;325:201–4. http://www.ncbi.nlm.nih.gov.

549. Colman RJ, Anderson RM, Johnson SC, et al. Caloric restriction delays disease onset and mortality in rhesus monkeys. *Science.* 2009;325(5937):201-4. http://www.ncbi.nlm.nih.gov.

550. Seyfried TN, Sanderson TM, El-Abbadi MM, McGowan R, Mukherjee P. Role of glucose and ketone bodies in the metabolic control of experimental brain

cancer. *Br J Cancer.* 2003;89:1375–1382.

551. Thammongkol S, Vears DF, Bicknell-Royle J, et al. Efficacy of the ketogenic diet: which epilepsies respond? *Epilepsia.* 2012;53(3):e55-9. http://www.ncbi.nlm.nih.gov.

552. Coppola G, Veggiotti P, Cusmai R, et al. The ketogenic diet in children, adolescents and young adults with refractory epilepsy: an Italian multicentric experience. *Epilepsy Res.* 2002;48(3):221-7. http://www.ncbi.nlm.nih.gov.

553. Sirven J, Whedon B, Caplan D, et al. The ketogenic diet for intractable epilepsy in adults: preliminary results. *Epilepsia.* 1999;40(12):1721-6. http://www.ncbi.nlm.nih.gov.

554. Kossoff EH, Thiele EA, Pfeifer HH, McGrogan JR, Freeman JM. Tuberous sclerosis complex and the ketogenic diet. *Epilepsia.* 2005;46(10):1684-6. http://www.ncbi.nlm.nih.gov.

555. Nebeling LC, Miraldi F, Shurin SB, Lerner E. Effects of a ketogenic diet on tumor metabolism and nutritional status in pediatric oncology patients: two case reports. *J Am Coll Nutr.* 1995;14(2):202-8. http://www.ncbi.nlm.nih.gov.

556. Swink TD, Vining EP, Freeman JM. The ketogenic diet:1997. *Adv Pediatr.* 1997;44:297-329. http://www.ncbi.nlm.nih.gov.

557. Mukherjee P, El-Abbadi MM, Kasperzyk JL, Ranes MK, Seyfried TN. Dietary restriction reduces angiogenesis and growth in an orthotopic mouse brain tumour model. *Br J Cancer.* 2002;86(10):1615-21. http://www.ncbi.nlm.nih.gov.

558. Seyfried TN, Marsh J, Shelton LM, Huysentruyt LC, Mukherjee P. Is the restricted ketogenic diet a viable alternative to the standard of care for managing malignant brain cancer? *Epilepsy Res. 2012;100(3):310-26.* http://www.ncbi.nlm.nih.gov.

559. Lee C, Longo VD. Fasting vs dietary restriction in cellular protection and cancer treatment: from model organisms to patients. *Oncogene.* 2011;30(30):3305-16. http://www.ncbi.nlm.nih.gov.

560. Lee C, Raffaghello L, Brandhorst S, et al. Fasting cycles retard growth of tumors and sensitize a range of cancer cell types to chemotherapy. *Sci Transl Med.* 2012;4(124):124ra27. http://www.ncbi.nlm.nih.gov.

561. Raffaghello L, et al. Starvation-dependent differential stress resistance protects normal but not cancer cells against high-dose chemotherapy. Proc Natl Acad Sci U S A. 2008;105(24):8215-20.

562. Lee C, Raffaghello L, Brandhorst S, et al. Fasting cycles retard growth of tumors and sensitize a range of cancer cell types to chemotherapy. *Sci Transl Med.* 2012;4(124):124ra27. http://www.ncbi.nlm.nih.gov.

563. Lee C. Reduced IGF-I differentially protects normal and cancer cells and improves chemotherapeutic index in mice. Cancer Res.2010; 70(4): 1564–1572.

564. Fernando M. Safdie, Tanya Dorff, David Quinn, Luigi Fontana, Min Wei, Changhan Lee, Pinchas Cohen, Valter D. Longo. Fasting and cancer treatment in humans: A case series report. *Aging (Albany NY)*. 2009; 1(12): 988–1007. http://www.ncbi.nlm.nih.gov.

565. Kenfield SA, Stampfer MJ, Giovannucci E, June M. Chan JM. Physical activity and survival after prostate cancer diagnosis in the health professionals follow-up study. *J Clin Oncol.* 2011; 29(6): 726–732. http://www.ncbi.nlm.nih.gov.

566. Barnard RJ, Ngo TH, Leung PS, Aronson WJ, Golding LA. A low-fat diet and/or strenuous exercise alters the IGF axis in vivo and reduces prostate tumor cell growth in vitro. *Prostate.* 2003;56(3):201-6. http://www.ncbi.nlm.nih.gov.

567. Leung PS, Aronson WJ, Ngo TH, et al. Exercise alters the IGF axis in vivo and increases p53 protein in prostate tumor cells in vitro. J Appl Physiol. 2004;96:450–454. http://www.ncbi.nlm.nih.gov.

568. Barnard RJ, Ngo TH, Leung PS, Aronson WJ, Golding LA. A low-fat diet and/or strenuous exercise alters the IGF axis in vivo and reduces prostate tumor cell growth in vitro. Prostate. 2003;56(3):201-6. http://www.ncbi.nlm.nih.gov.

569. Yang D, Bernstein L, Wu AH. Physical activity and breast cancer risk among Asian-American women in Los Angeles: a case-control study. *Cancer.* 2003;97(10):2565-75. http://www.ncbi.nlm.nih.gov.

570. Bernstein L, Patel AV, Ursin G, et al. Lifetime recreational exercise activity and breast cancer risk among black women and white women. *J Natl Cancer Inst.* 2005;97(22):1671. http://www.ncbi.nlm.nih.gov.

571. John EM, Horn-Ross PL, Koo J. Lifetime physical activity and breast cancer risk in a multiethnic population: the San Francisco Bay area breast cancer study. *Cancer Epidemiol Biomarkers Prev.* 2003;12(11 Pt 1):1143-52. http://www.ncbi.nlm.nih.gov.

572. Kruk J. Lifetime physical activity and the risk of breast cancer: a case-control study. *Cancer Detect Prev.* 2007;31(1):18-28. http://www.ncbi.nlm.nih.gov.

573. Patel AV, Press MF, Meeske K, Calle EE, Bernstein L. Lifetime recreational exercise activity and risk of breast carcinoma in situ. *Cancer.* 2003;98(10):2161-9. http://www.ncbi.nlm.nih.gov.

574. Verloop J, Rookus MA, Kooy K, Leeuwen FE. Physical activity and breast cancer risk in women aged 20-54 years. *J Natl Cancer Inst.*1999;92(2):128-135. http://www.ncbi.nlm.nih.gov.

575. Kossman DA, Williams NI, Domchek SM, Kurzer MS, Stopfer JE, Schmitz KH. Exercise lowers estrogen and progesterone levels in premenopausal women at high risk of breast cancer. *J Appl Physiol.* 2011;111(6):1687-93. http://www.ncbi.nlm.nih.gov.

576. Bertram LA, Stefanick ML, Saquib N, et al. Physical activity, additional breast cancer events, and mortality among early-stage breast cancer survivors: find-

ings from the WHEL Study. *Cancer Causes Control.* 2011;22(3):427-35.

577. Saquib N, Pierce JP, Saquib J, et. al. Poor physical health predicts time to additional breast cancer events and mortality in breast cancer survivors. *Psychooncology.* 2011;20(3):252-9.

578. Kenfield SA, Stampfer MJ, Giovannucci E, Chan JM. Physical Activity and Survival After Prostate Cancer Diagnosis in the Health Professionals Follow-Up Study. *J Clin Oncol.* 2011;29(6):726-32. http://www.ncbi.nlm.nih.gov.

579. Wolin KY, Yan Y, Colditz GA. Physical activity and risk of colon adenoma: a meta-analysis. *Br J Cancer.* 2011; 104(5): 882–885. http://www.ncbi.nlm.nih.gov.

580. Sanchez NF, Bryan Stierman B, Saab S, et al. Physical activity reduces risk for colon polyps in a multiethnic colorectal cancer screening population. *BMC Res Notes.* 2012;5:312.

581. Zhang J, Dhakal IB, Gross MD, et al. Physical Activity, Diet, and Pancreatic Cancer: A Population-Based Case-Control Study in Minnesota. *Nutr Cancer. 2009;* 61(4): 457–465. http://www.ncbi.nlm.nih.gov.

582. Michaud DS, Giovannucci E, Willett WC, Colditz GA, Stampfer MJ, Fuchs CS. Physical activity, obesity, height, and the risk of pancreatic cancer. *JAMA.* 2001;286(8):921-9. http://www.ncbi.nlm.nih.gov.

583. Calton BA, Stolzenberg-Solomon RZ, Moore SC, et al. A prospective study of physical activity and the risk of pancreatic cancer among women (United States). *BMC Cancer.* 2008;8:63.

584. Moore SC, Gierach GL, Schatzkin A, Matthews CE. Physical activity, sedentary behaviours, and the prevention of endometrial cancer. *Br J Cancer.* 2010; 103(7): 933–938. http://www.ncbi.nlm.nih.gov.

585. Gierach GL, Chang SC, Brinton LA, et al. Physical Activity, Sedentary Behavior, and Endometrial Cancer Risk in the NIH-AARP Diet and Health Study. *Int J Cancer.* 20091; 124(9): 2139–2147.

586. Buffart LM, Singh AS, van Loon EC, Vermeulen HI, Brug J, Chinapaw MJ. Physical activity and the risk of developing lung cancer among smokers: A meta-analysis. *J Sci Med Sport.* 2013; S1440-2440(13)00047-9.

587. Sun JY, Shi L, Gao XD, Xu SF. Physical activity and risk of lung cancer: a meta-analysis of Prospective Cohort Studies. *Asian Pac J Cancer Prev.* 2012;13(7):3143-7. http://www.ncbi.nlm.nih.gov.

588. Sun JY, Shi L, Gao XD, Xu SF. Physical activity and risk of lung cancer: a meta-analysis of Prospective Cohort Studies. *Asian Pac J Cancer Prev.* 2012;13(7):3143-7. http://www.ncbi.nlm.nih.gov.

589. Zucker D. *Cancer and Obesity:* The role exercise plays in cancer treatment. May 12, 2012. Swedish Cancer Institute. http://www.swedish.org.

590. AICR'S foods that fight cancer. American Institute for Cancer Research; 2014. http://www.aicr.org

591. Doll R, Peto R. The causes of cancer. Quantitative estimates of avoidable risks of cancer in the United States today. *J Natl Cancer Inst.* 1981;66:1193–1208. http://www.ncbi.nlm.nih.gov.

592. Food, Nutrition, Physical Activity, and the Prevention of Cancer: a Global Perspective. American Institute for Cancer Research; 2007. http://www.aicr.org.

593. Levi F, Pasche C, La Vecchia C, Lucchini F, Franceschi S, Monnier P. Food groups and risk of oral and pharyngeal cancer. *Int J Cancer.* 1998;77(5):705-9. http://www.ncbi.nlm.nih.gov.

594. Johnson CM, Wei C, Ensor JE, et al. Meta-analyses of colorectal cancer risk factors. *Cancer Causes Control. 2013;*24(6):1207-22. http://www.ncbi.nlm.nih.gov.

595. Ashmore JH, Lesko SM, Miller PE, et al. Association of dietary and supplemental iron and colorectal cancer in a population-based study. *Eur J Cancer Prev.* 2013;22(6):506-11. http://www.ncbi.nlm.nih.gov.

596. Chao A, Thun MJ, Connell CJ, McCullough ML, Jacobs EJ, Flanders WD, Rodriguez C, Sinha R, Calle EE. Meat consumption and risk of colorectal cancer. *JAMA.* 2005;293(2):172-182. http://www.ncbi.nlm.nih.gov.

597. Giovannucci E, Rimm EB, Stampfer MJ, Colditz GA, Ascherio A, Willett WC. Intake of fat, meat, and fiber in relation to risk of colon cancer in men. *Cancer Res.* 1994;54(9):2390-7.

598. Willett WC, Stampfer MJ, Colditz GA, Rosner BA, Speizer FE. Relation of meat, fat, and fiber intake to the risk of colon cancer in a prospective study among women. *N Engl J Med.* 1990;323(24):1664-72. http://www.ncbi.nlm.nih.gov.

599. Rohrmann S, Platz EA, Kavanaugh CJ, Thuita L, Hoffman SC, Helzlsouer KJ. Meat and dairy consumption and subsequent risk of prostate cancer in a US cohort study. *Cancer Causes Control.* 2007;18(1):41-50. http://www.ncbi.nlm.nih.gov.

600. Rodriguez C, McCullough ML, Mondul AM, et al. Meat consumption among Black and White men and risk of prostate cancer in the Cancer Prevention Study II Nutrition Cohort. *Cancer Epidemiol Biomarkers Prev.* 2006;15(2):211-6. http://www.ncbi.nlm.nih.gov.

601. Larsson SC, Wolk A. Red and processed meat consumption and risk of pancreatic cancer: meta-analysis of prospective studies. Br J Cancer. 2012;106(3):603-7. http://www.ncbi.nlm.nih.gov.

602. Bao PP, Shu XO, Zheng Y, et al. Fruit, vegetable, and animal food intake and breast cancer risk by hormone receptor status. *Nutr Cancer.* 2012;64(6):806-19. http://www.ncbi.nlm.nih.gov.

603. Fu Z, Deming SL, Fair AM, Shrubsole MJ, Wujcik DM, Shu XO, Kelley M, Zheng W. Well-done meat intake and meat-derived mutagen exposures in rela-

tion to breast cancer risk: the Nashville Breast Health Study. *Breast Cancer Res Treat.* 2011;129(3):919-28.

604. Cho E, Spiegelman D, Hunter DJ, Chen WY, Stampfer MJ, Colditz GA, Willett WC. Premenopausal fat intake and risk of breast cancer. *J Natl Cancer Inst.* 2003;95(14):1079-85. http://www.ncbi.nlm.nih.gov.

605. Boyd NF, Stone J, Vogt KN, Connelly BS, Martin LJ, Minkin S. Dietary fat and breast cancer risk revisited: a meta-analysis of the published literature. *Br J Cancer.* 2003;89(9):1672-85. http://www.ncbi.nlm.nih.gov.

606. Ward MH, Cross AJ, Abnet CC, Sinha R, Markin RS, Weisenburger DD. Heme iron from meat and risk of adenocarcinoma of the esophagus and stomach. *Eur J Cancer Prev.* 2012;21(2):134-8. http://www.ncbi.nlm.nih.gov.

607. van Lonkhuijzen L, Kirsh VA, Kreiger N, Rohan TE. Endometrial cancer and meat consumption: a case-cohort study. *Eur J Cancer Prev.* 2011;20(4):334-9. http://www.ncbi.nlm.nih.gov.

608. Kallianpur AR, Lee SA, Xu WH, et al. Dietary iron intake and risk of endometrial cancer: a population-based case-control study in Shanghai, China. *Nutr Cancer.* 2010;62(1):40-50. http://www.ncbi.nlm.nih.gov.

609. Bandera EV, Kushi LH, Moore DF, Gifkins DM, McCullough ML. Consumption of animal foods and endometrial cancer risk: a systematic literature review and meta-analysis. *Cancer Causes Control.* 2007;18(9):967-88. http://www.ncbi.nlm.nih.gov.

610. Keszei AP, Schouten LJ, Goldbohm RA, van den Brandt PA. Red and processed meat consumption and the risk of esophageal and gastric cancer subtypes in The Netherlands Cohort Study. *Ann Oncol.* 2012;23(9):2319-26. http://www.ncbi.nlm.nih.gov.

611. Cross AJ, Freedman ND, Ren J, Ward MH, Hollenbeck AR, Schatzkin A, Sinha R, Abnet CC. Meat consumption and risk of esophageal and gastric cancer in a large prospective study. *Am J Gastroenterol. 2011;106(3):432-42.* http://www.ncbi.nlm.nih.gov.

612. De Stefani E, Boffetta P, Ronco AL, et al. Processed meat consumption and risk of cancer: a multisite case-control study in Uruguay. *Br J Cancer.* 2012;107(9):1584-8. http://www.ncbi.nlm.nih.gov.

613. Ward MH, Cross AJ, Abnet CC, Sinha R, Markin RS, Weisenburger DD. Heme iron from meat and risk of adenocarcinoma of the esophagus and stomach. *Eur J Cancer Prev.* 2012;21(2):134-8. http://www.ncbi.nlm.nih.gov.

614. Jakszyn P, Agudo A, Lujan-Barroso L, et al. Dietary intake of heme iron and risk of gastric cancer in the European prospective investigation into cancer and nutrition study. *Int J Cancer.* 2012;130(11):2654-63. http://www.ncbi.nlm.nih.gov.

615. Hu J, La Vecchia C, Morrison H, et al. Salt, processed meat and the risk of cancer. *Eur J Cancer Prev.* 2011(2):132-9. http://www.ncbi.nlm.nih.gov.

616. Aune D, De Stefani E, Ronco A, et al. Meat consumption and cancer risk: a case-control study in Uruguay. *Asian Pac J Cancer Prev.* 2009;10(3):429-36. http://www.ncbi.nlm.nih.gov.

617. Fontana L, Adelaiye RM, Rastelli AL, et al. Dietary protein restriction inhibits tumor growth in human xenograft models of prostate and breast cancer. Oncotarget. 2013;4(12):2451-61. http://www.ncbi.nlm.nih.gov.

618. Turner LB. A meta-analysis of fat intake, reproduction, and breast cancer risk: an evolutionary perspective. *Am J Hum Biol.* 2011;23(5):601-8. http://www.ncbi.nlm.nih.gov.

619. Boyd NF, Stone J, Vogt KN, Connelly BS, Martin LJ, Minkin S. Dietary fat and breast cancer risk revisited: a meta-analysis of the published literature. *Br J Cancer.* 2003;89(9):1672-85. http://www.ncbi.nlm.nih.gov.

620. Rose DP, Boyar AP, Cohen C, Strong LE. Effect of a low-fat diet on hormone levels in women with cystic breast disease. I. Serum steroids and gonadotropins. *J Natl Cancer Inst.* 1987;78(4):623-6. http://www.ncbi.nlm.nih.gov.

621. Wu AH, Pike MC, Stram DO. Meta-analysis: dietary fat intake, serum estrogen levels, and the risk of breast cancer. *Am J Ind Med.* 2010;53(12):1197-206. http://www.ncbi.nlm.nih.gov.

622. Ingram DM, Bennett FC, Willcox D, de Klerk N. Effect of low-fat diet on female sex hormone levels. *J Natl Cancer Inst.* 1987;79(6):1225-9. http://www.ncbi.nlm.nih.gov.

623. Ingram DM, Bennett FC, Willcox D, de Klerk N. Effect of low-fat diet on female sex hormone levels. *J Natl Cancer Inst.* 1987;79(6):1225-9. http://www.ncbi.nlm.nih.gov.

624. Cho E, Spiegelman D, Hunter DJ, Chen WY, Stampfer MJ, Colditz GA, Willett WC. Premenopausal fat intake and risk of breast cancer. *J Natl Cancer Inst.* 2003;95(14):1079-85. http://www.ncbi.nlm.nih.gov.

625. Dong JY, Zhang L, He K, Qin LQ. Dairy consumption and risk of breast cancer: a meta-analysis of prospective cohort studies. *Breast Cancer Res Treat.* 2011;127(1):23-31. http://www.ncbi.nlm.nih.gov.

626. Kesse-Guyot E, Bertrais S, Duperray B, et al. Dairy products, calcium and the risk of breast cancer: results of the French SU.VI.MAX prospective study. *Ann Nutr Metab.* 2007;51(2):139-45. http://www.ncbi.nlm.nih.gov.

627. Ganmaa D, Sato A. The possible role of female sex hormones in milk from pregnant cows in the development of breast, ovarian and corpus uteri cancers. *Med Hypotheses.* 2005;65(6):1028-37. http://www.ncbi.nlm.nih.gov.

628. Shin MH, Holmes MD, Hankinson SE, Wu K, Colditz GA, Willett WC. Intake of dairy products, calcium, and vitamin d and risk of breast cancer. *J Natl Can-*

cer Inst. 2002;94(17):1301-11. http://www.ncbi.nlm.nih.gov.

629. Kroenke CH, Kwan ML, Sweeney C, Castillo A, Caan BJ. High- and low-fat dairy intake, recurrence, and mortality after breast cancer diagnosis. *J Natl Cancer Inst.* 2013;105(9):616-23. http://www.ncbi.nlm.nih.gov.

630. Trock BJ, Hilakivi-Clarke L, Clarke R. Meta-analysis of soy intake and breast cancer risk. *J Natl Cancer Inst.* 2006;98(7):459-71. http://www.ncbi.nlm.nih.gov.

631. Sarkar FH, Li Y. Soy isoflavones and cancer prevention. *Cancer Invest.* 2003;21(5):744-57. http://www.ncbi.nlm.nih.gov.

632. Lamartiniere CA, Moore JB, Brown NM, et al. Genistein suppresses mammary cancer in rats. *Carcinogenesis.* 1995;16(11):2833-40. http://www.ncbi.nlm.nih.gov.

633. Allred CD, Ju YH, Allred KF, Chang J, Helferich WG. Dietary genistin stimulates growth of estrogen-dependent breast cancer tumors similar to that observed with genistein. *Carcinogenesis.* 2001;22(10):1667-73. http://www.ncbi.nlm.nih.gov.

634. Allred CD, Allred KF, Ju YH, et al. Dietary genistein results in larger MNU-induced, estrogen-dependent mammary tumors following ovariectomy of Sprague-Dawley rats. *Carcinogenesis.* 2004;25(2):211–8. http://www.ncbi.nlm.nih.gov.

635. De Lemos ML. Effects of soy phytoestrogens genistein and daidzein on breast cancer growth. *Ann Pharmacother.* 2001;35(9):1118-21. http://www.ncbi.nlm.nih.gov.

636. Tomar RS, Shiao R. Early life and adult exposure to isoflavones and breast cancer risk. *J Environ Sci Health C Environ Carcinog Ecotoxicol Rev.* 2008;26(2):113-73. http://www.ncbi.nlm.nih.gov.

637. Lamartiniere CA. Protection against breast cancer with genistein: a component of soy. *Am J Clin Nutr. 200071(6 Suppl):1705S-7S.* http://www.ncbi.nlm.nih.gov.

638. Fritz W. A., Coward L., Wang J., Lamartiniere C. A. Dietary genistein: perinatal mammary cancer prevention, bioavailability and toxicity testing in the rat. *Carcinogenesis (Lond) 1998;*19:2151-2158. http://www.ncbi.nlm.nih.gov.

639. Lamartiniere C. A., Moore J. B., Brown N. M., et al. Genistein suppresses mammary cancer in rats. *Carcinogenesis (Lond)1996;* 16:2833-2840. http://www.ncbi.nlm.nih.gov.

640. Murrill W. B., Brown N. M., Zhang J. X., et al. Prepubertal genistein exposure suppresses mammary cancer and enhances gland differentiation in rats. *Carcinogenesis (Lond). 1996;17:1451-1457.* http://www.ncbi.nlm.nih.gov.

641. Rowell C, Carpenter DM, Lamartiniere CA. Chemoprevention of breast cancer, proteomic discovery of genistein action in the rat mammary gland. *J Nutr.*

2005;135(12 Suppl):2953S-2959S. http://www.ncbi.nlm.nih.gov.

642. Lee SA, Shu XO, Li H, et al. Adolescent and adult soy food intake and breast cancer risk: results from the Shanghai Women's Health Study. *Am J Clin Nutr.* 2009;89(6):1920-6. http://www.ncbi.nlm.nih.gov.

643. Shu XO, Zheng Y, Cai H, Gu K, Chen Z, Zheng W, Lu W. Soy food intake and breast cancer survival. *JAMA. 2009;302(22):2437-43.* http://www.ncbi.nlm.nih.gov.

644. Kang HB, Zhang YF, Yang JD, Lu KL. Study on soy isoflavone consumption and risk of breast cancer and survival. *Asian Pac J Cancer Prev.* 2012;13(3):995-8. http://www.ncbi.nlm.nih.gov.

645. Caan BJ, Natarajan L, Parker B, et al. Soy food consumption and breast cancer prognosis. *Cancer Epidemiol Biomarkers Prev.* 2011;20(5):854-8. http://www.ncbi.nlm.nih.gov.

646. Magee PJ, Rowland I. Soy products in the management of breast cancer. *Curr Opin Clin Nutr Metab Care. 2012;15(6):586-91.* http://www.ncbi.nlm.nih.gov.

647. Dong JY, Qin LQ. Soy isoflavones consumption and risk of breast cancer incidence or recurrence: a meta-analysis of prospective studies. *Breast Cancer Res Treat.* 2011;125(2):315-23. http://www.ncbi.nlm.nih.gov.

648. Khan SA, Chatterton RT, Michel N, et al. Soy Isoflavone supplementation for breast cancer risk reduction: a randomized phase II trial. *Cancer Prev Res (Phila).* 2012;5(2):309-19.

649. Berryman CE, Grieger JA, West SG, et al. Acute Consumption of Walnuts and Walnut Components Differentially Affect Postprandial Lipemia, Endothelial Function, Oxidative Stress, and Cholesterol Efflux in Humans with Mild Hypercholesterolemia. *J Nutr. 2013*;143(6):788-94. http://www.ncbi.nlm.nih.gov.

650. Pan A, Sun Q, Manson JE, Willett WC, Hu FB. Walnut consumption is associated with lower risk of type 2 diabetes in women. *J Nutr.* 2013;143(4):512-8. http://www.ncbi.nlm.nih.gov.

651. Hardman WE, Ion G, Akinsete JA, Witte TR. Dietary walnut suppressed mammary gland tumorigenesis in the C(3)1 TAg mouse. *Nutr Cancer.* 2011;63(6):960-70. http://www.ncbi.nlm.nih.gov.

652. Vanden Heuvel JP, Belda BJ, Hannon DB, et al. Mechanistic examination of walnuts in prevention of breast cancer. *Nutr Cancer.* 2012;64(7):1078-86. http://www.ncbi.nlm.nih.gov.

653. Hardman WE, Ion G. Suppression of implanted MDA-MB 231 human breast cancer growth in nude mice by dietary walnut. *Nutr Cancer.* 2008;60(5):666-74. http://www.ncbi.nlm.nih.gov.

654. Davis PA, Vasu VT, Gohil K, et al. A high-fat diet containing whole walnuts (Juglans regia) reduces tumour size and growth along with plasma insulin-

like growth factor 1 in the transgenic adenocarcinoma of the mouse prostate model. *Br J Nutr.* 2012;108(10):1764-72. http://www.ncbi.nlm.nih.gov.

655. Nagel JM, Brinkoetter M, Magkos F, et al. Dietary walnuts inhibit colorectal cancer growth in mice by suppressing angiogenesis. *Nutrition.* 2012;28(1):67-75. http://www.ncbi.nlm.nih.gov.

656. Sherman ME, Figueroa JD, Henry JE, et al. The Susan G. Komen for the Cure Tissue Bank at the IU Simon Cancer Center: a unique resource for defining the "molecular histology" of the breast. Cancer Prev Res.2012;5(4):528–535. http://www.ncbi.nlm.nih.gov.

657. Forster N, Saladi SV, van Bragt M, Sfondouris ME, Jones FE, Li Z, Ellisen LW. Basal Cell Signaling by p63 Controls Luminal Progenitor Function and Lactation via NRG1. Dev Cell. 2014;28(2):147-60. http://www.ncbi.nlm.nih.gov.

658. Taylor-Papadimitriou J, Berdichevsky F, D'Souza B, Burchell J. Human models of breast cancer. Cancer Surv.1993;16:59-78. http://www.ncbi.nlm.nih.gov.

659. Silanikove N. Natural and abrupt involution of the mammary gland affects differently the metabolic and health consequences of weaning. Life Sci. 2014; pii: S0024-3205(14)00291-4. http://www.ncbi.nlm.nih.gov.

660. Baltzer A, Svanborg C, Jaggi R. Apoptotic cell death in the lactating mammary gland is enhanced by a folding variant of alpha-lactalbumin. Cell Mol Life Sci. 2004;61(10):1221-8. http://www.ncbi.nlm.nih.gov.

661. Stein T, Salomonis N, Gusterson BA. Mammary gland involution as a multi-step process. J Mammary Gland Biol Neoplasia. 2007;12(1):25-35. http://www.ncbi.nlm.nih.gov.

662. Wilde CJ, Knight CH, Flint DJ. Control of milk secretion and apoptosis during mammary involution. J Mammary Gland Biol Neoplasia. 1999;4(2):129-36. http://www.ncbi.nlm.nih.gov.

663. CJ, Watson. Involution: apoptosis and tissue remodelling that convert the mammary gland from milk factory to a quiescent organ. Breast Cancer Research. 2006;8(2):203. http://www.ncbi.nlm.nih.gov.

664. Breastfeeding. Switzerland:World Health Organization;2014. http://www.who.int.org.

665. Gajalakshmi V, Mathew A, Brennan P, et al. Breastfeeding and breast cancer risk in India: a multicenter case-control study. J Cancer. 2009;125(3):662-5. http://www.ncbi.nlm.nih.gov.

666. Layde PM, Webster LA, Baughman AL, Wingo PA, Rubin GL, Ory HW. The independent associations of parity, age at first full term pregnancy, and

duration of breastfeeding with the risk of breast cancer. Cancer and Steroid Hormone Study Group. J Clin Epidemiol. 1989;42(10):963-73. http://www.ncbi.nlm.nih.gov.

667. McTiernan A, Thomas DB. Evidence for a protective effect of lactation on risk of breast cancer in young women. Results from a case-control study. Am J Epidemiol. 1986;124(3):353-8. http://www.ncbi.nlm.nih.gov.

668. Newcomb PA, Storer BE, Longnecker MP, Lactation and a reduced risk of premenopausal breast cancer. N Engl J Med.1994;330(2):81-7. http://www.ncbi.nlm.nih.gov.

669. Yoo KY, Tajima K, Kuroishi T, Hirose K, Yoshida M, Miura S, Murai H.Independent protective effect of lactation against breast cancer: a case-control study in Japan. Am J Epidemiol. 1992;135(7):726-33. http://www.ncbi.nlm.nih.gov.

670. Romieu I, Hernández-Avila M, Lazcano E, Lopez L, Romero-Jaime R. Breast cancer and lactation history in Mexican women. Am J Epidemiol. 1996;143(6):543-52. http://www.ncbi.nlm.nih.gov.

671. Kim Y, Choi JY, Lee KM, et al. Dose-dependent protective effect of breastfeeding against breast cancer among ever-lactated women in Korea. Eur J Cancer Prev. 2007;16(2):124-9. http://www.ncbi.nlm.nih.gov.

672. Awatef M, Olfa G, Imed H, Kacem M, Imen C, Rim C, Mohamed B, Slim BA.Breastfeeding reduces breast cancer risk: a case-control study in Tunisia. Cancer Causes Control. 2010;;21(3):393-7. http://www.ncbi.nlm.nih.gov.

673. Tryggvadóttir L, Tulinius H, Eyfjord JE, Sigurvinsson T.Breastfeeding and reduced risk of breast cancer in an Icelandic cohort study. Am J Epidemiol. 2001;154(1):37-42. http://www.ncbi.nlm.nih.gov.

674. Chie W, Lee W, Li C, Huang C, Chang K, Yen M, Lin R.Lactation, lactation suppression hormones and breast cancer. Oncol Rep. 1997;4(2):319-26.

675. Collaborative Group on Hormonal Factors in Breast Cancer.Breast cancer and breastfeeding: collaborative reanalysis of individual data from 47 epidemiological studies in 30 countries, including 50302 women with breast cancer and 96973 women without the disease. Lancet. 2002;360(9328):187-95. http://www.ncbi.nlm.nih.gov.

676. Table 2: Nutrition. New York: UNICEF;2003.www.http://www.unicef.org.

677. Nutrition in the first 1000 days: 13th annual state of the world mothers: The infant and toddler feeding scorecard. Westport, CT:Save the children; 2012. http://www.savethechildren.

678. Breast cancer incidence worldwide. Dallas, TX: Susan G. Komen;2012. http://ww5.komen.org.

679. Ferlay J, Soerjomataram I, Ervik M, et al. Globocan 2012 v1.0, Cancer Incidence and Mortality Worldwide: IARC CancerBase No. 11. Lyon, France: International Agency for Research on Cancer; 2013.

680. Shetty P. India faces growing breast cancer epidemic. Lancet. 2012;379(9820):992-3. http://www.ncbi.nlm.nih.gov.

681. Carruba G. Estrogens and mechanisms of prostate cancer progression. *Ann N Y Acad Sci.* 2006;1089:201-17. http://www.ncbi.nlm.nih.gov.

682. Abd Elmageed ZY, Moroz K, Srivastav SK, et al. High Circulating Estrogens and Selective Expression of ERβ in Prostate Tumors: Implications for Racial Disparity of Prostate Cancer. *Carcinogenesis.* 2013;34(9):2017-23. http://www.ncbi.nlm.nih.gov.

683. Prins GS, Korach KS. The Role of Estrogens and Estrogen Receptors in Normal Prostate Growth and Disease. *Steroids.* 2008;73(3):233-44. http://www.ncbi.nlm.nih.gov.

684. Lophatananon A, Archer J, Easton D, et al. Dietary fat and early-onset prostate cancer risk. *Br J Nutr.* 2010;103(9):1375-80. http://www.ncbi.nlm.nih.gov.

685. Lophatananon A, Archer J, Easton D, et al. Dietary fat and early-onset prostate cancer. Dietary fat and early-onset prostate cancer risk. *Br J Nutr.* 2010;103(9):1375-80. http://www.ncbi.nlm.nih.gov.

686. Giovannucci E, Rimm EB, Colditz GA, Stampfer MJ, Ascherio A, Chute CC, Willett WC. A prospective study of dietary fat and risk of prostate cancer. *J Natl Cancer Inst.* 1993;85(19):1571-9. http://www.ncbi.nlm.nih.gov.

687. Rohrmann S, Platz EA, Kavanaugh CJ, Thuita L, Hoffman SC, Helzlsouer KJ. Meat and dairy consumption and subsequent risk of prostate cancer in a US cohort study. *Cancer Causes Control.* 2007;18(1):41-50. http://www.ncbi.nlm.nih.gov.

688. Michaud DS, Augustsson K, Rimm EB, Stampfer MJ, Willet WC, Giovannucci E. A prospective study on intake of animal products and risk of prostate cancer. *Cancer Causes Control.* 2001;12(6):557-67. http://www.ncbi.nlm.nih.gov.

689. Rodriguez C, McCullough ML, Mondul AM, Jacobs EJ, Chao A, et al. Greater consumption of fat from animal sources to increased risk for prostate cancer among American blacks. *Cancer Epidemiol Biomarkers Prev.* 2006;15:211–216. http://www.ncbi.nlm.nih.gov.

690. -Hayes RB, Ziegler RG, Gridley G, et al. Dietary factors and risks for prostate cancer among blacks and whites in the United States. *Cancer Epidemiol Biomarkers Prev.* 1999;8(1):25-34. http://www.ncbi.nlm.nih.gov.

691. Cross AJ, Sinha R. Meat-related mutagens/carcinogens in the etiology of colorectal cancer. *Environmental and Molecular Mutagenesis.* 2004; 44(1):44–

55. http://www.ncbi.nlm.nih.gov.

692. John EM, Stern MC, Sinha R, KooJ. Meat consumption, Cooking Practices, Meat Mutagens and Risk of Prostate Cancer. *Nutr Cancer.* 2011; 63(4): 525–537. http://www.ncbi.nlm.nih.gov.

693. Cross AJ, Peters U, Kirsh VA, Andriole GL, Reding D, Hayes RB, Sinha R. A prospective study of meat and meat mutagens and prostate cancer risk. *Cancer Res.* 2005;65(24):11779-84. http://www.ncbi.nlm.nih.gov.

694. Koutros S, Cross AJ, Sandler DP, Hoppin JA, Ma X, Zheng T, Alavanja MC, Sinha R. Meat and meat mutagens and risk of prostate cancer in the Agricultural Health Study. *Cancer Epidemiol Biomarkers Prev.* 2008;17(1):80-7. http://www.ncbi.nlm.nih.gov.

695. Norrish AE, Ferguson LR, Knize MG, Felton JS, Sharpe SJ, Jackson RT. Heterocyclic amine content of cooked meat and risk of prostate cancer. *J Natl Cancer Inst.* 19991;91(23):2038-44. http://www.ncbi.nlm.nih.gov.

696. Kato T, Ohgaki H, Hasegawa H, et al. Carcinogenicity in rats of a mutagenic compound, 2-amino-3,8-dimethylimidazo[4,5-f]quinoxaline. *Carcinogenesis.* 1988; 9(1):71–73. http://www.ncbi.nlm.nih.gov.

697. Committee on Diet, Nutrition, and Cancer. Diet, Nutrition and Cancer. National Academy Press, Washington DC; 1982. http://nap.edu.

698. Punnen S, Hardin J, Cheng I, Klein EA, Witte JS. Impact of meat consumption, preparation, and mutagens on aggressive prostate cancer. *PLoS One.* 2011;6(11):e27711. http://www.ncbi.nlm.nih.gov.

699. Major JM, Cross AJ, et al. Patterns of meat intake and risk of prostate cancer among African-Americans in a large prospective cohort of men. *Cancer Causes Control. 2011;* 22(12): 1691–1698. http://www.ncbi.nlm.nih.gov.

700. Michaud DS, Augustsson K, Rimm EB, Stampfer MJ, Willet WC, Giovannucci E.A prospective study on intake of animal products and risk of prostate cancer. Cancer Causes Control. 2001;12(6):557-67.

701. Qin LQ, Wang PY, Kaneko T, Hoshi K, Sato A. Estrogen: one of the risk factors in milk for prostate cancer. *Med Hypotheses.* 2004;62(1):133-42. http://www.ncbi.nlm.nih.gov.

702. Qin LQ, Xu JY, Wang PY, Tong J, Hoshi K. Milk consumption is a risk factor for prostate cancer in Western countries: evidence from cohort studies. *Asia Pac J Clin Nutr.* 2007;16(3):467-76. http://www.ncbi.nlm.nih.gov.

703. Chan JM, Stampfer MJ, Ma J, Gann PH, Gaziano JM, Giovannucci EL. Dairy products, calcium, and prostate cancer risk in the Physicians' Health Study. *Am J Clin Nutr.* 2001;74(4):549-54. http://www.ncbi.nlm.nih.gov.

704. Melnik BC, John SM, Carrera-Bastos P, Cordain L. The impact of cow's milk-mediated mTORC1-signaling in the initiation and progression of prostate

cancer. *Nutr Metab (Lond).* 2012;9(1):74. http://www.ncbi.nlm.nih.gov.

705. Chan JM, Giovannucci E, Andersson SO, Yuen J, Adami HO, Wolk A. Dairy products, calcium, phosphorous, vitamin D, and risk of prostate cancer (Sweden). *Cancer Causes Control.* 1998;9(6):559-66. http://www.ncbi.nlm.nih.gov.

706. Rock CL. Milk and the risk and progression of cancer. *Nestle Nutr Workshop Ser Pediatr Program.* 2011;67:173-85. http://www.ncbi.nlm.nih.gov.

707. Tate PL, Bibb R, Larcom LL. Milk stimulates growth of prostate cancer cells in culture. *Nutr Cancer.* 2011;63(8):1361-6. http://www.ncbi.nlm.nih.gov.

708. Giovannucci E, Liu Y, Stampfer MJ, Willett WC. A prospective study of calcium intake and incident and fatal prostate cancer. *Cancer Epidemiol Biomarkers Prev.* 2006;15(2):203-10. http://www.ncbi.nlm.nih.gov.

709. Park Y, Mitrou PN, Kipnis V, Hollenbeck A, Schatzkin A, Leitzmann MF. Calcium, dairy 68, and risk of incident and fatal prostate cancer: the NIH-AARP Diet and Health Study. *Am J Epidemiol.* 2007;166(11):1270-9. http://www.ncbi.nlm.nih.gov.

710. Giovannucci E, Liu Y, Stampfer MJ, Willett WC. A prospective study of calcium intake and incident and fatal prostate cancer. *Cancer Epidemiol Biomarkers Prev.* 2006;15(2):203-10. http://www.ncbi.nlm.nih.gov.

711. Song Y, Chavarro JE, Cao Y, et al. Whole milk intake is associated with prostate cancer-specific mortality among U.S. male physicians. *J Nutr.* 2013; 143(2):189-96.

712. Park Y, Mitrou PN, Kipnis V, Hollenbeck A, Schatzkin A, Leitzmann MF. Calcium, dairy foods, and risk of incident and fatal prostate cancer: the NIH-AARP Diet and Health Study. *Am J Epidemiol.* 2007;166(11):1270-9. http://www.ncbi.nlm.nih.gov.

713. Tate PL, Bibb R, Larcom LL. Milk stimulates growth of prostate cancer cells in culture. *Nutr Cancer.* 2011;63(8):1361-6. http://www.ncbi.nlm.nih.gov.

714. Hwang YW, Kim SY, Jee SH, Kim YN, Nam CM. Soy food consumption and risk of prostate cancer: a meta-analysis of observational studies. *Nutr Cancer.* 2009;61(5):598-606. http://www.ncbi.nlm.nih.gov.

715. Yan L, Spitznagel EL. Soy consumption and prostate cancer risk in men: a revisit of a meta-analysis. *Am J Clin Nutr.* 2009;89(4):1155-63. http://www.ncbi.nlm.nih.gov.

716. Hwang YW, Kim SY, Jee SH, Kim YN, Nam CM. Soy food consumption and risk of prostate cancer: a meta-analysis of observational studies. *Nutr Cancer.* 2009;61(5):598-606. http://www.ncbi.nlm.nih.gov.

717. Hamilton-Reeves JM, Rebello SA, Thomas W, Slaton JW, Kurzer MS. Soy protein isolate 69 urinary estrogens and the ratio of 2:16alpha-hydroxyestrone

in men at high risk of prostate cancer. *J Nutr.* 2007;137(10):2258-63. http://www.ncbi.nlm.nih.gov.

718. Hamilton-Reeves JM, Rebello SA, Thomas W, Slaton JW, Kurzer MS. Isoflavone-rich soy protein isolate suppresses androgen receptor expression without altering estrogen receptor-beta expression or serum hormonal profiles in men at high risk of prostate cancer. *J Nutr.* 2007;137(7):1769-75. http://www.ncbi.nlm.nih.gov.
719. Pantuck AJ, Leppert JT, Zomorodian N, et al. Phase II study of pomegranate juice for men with rising prostate-specific antigen following surgery or radiation for prostate cancer. *Clinical Cancer Research.* 2006;12(13):4018–4026. http://www.ncbi.nlm.nih.gov.
720. Forest CP, Padma-Nathan H, Liker HR. Efficacy and safety of pomegranate juice on improvement of erectile dysfunction in male patients with mild to moderate erectile dysfunction: a randomized, placebo-controlled, double-blind, crossover study. Int J Impot Res. 2007;19(6):564–567.
721. Kroeger N, Belldegrun AS, Pantuck AJ . Pomegranate Extracts in the Management of Men's Urologic Health: Scientific Rationale and Preclinical and Clinical Data. *Evid Based Complement Alternat Med.* 2013;2013:701434. http://www.ncbi.nlm.nih.gov.
722. Pantuck AJ, Leppert JT, Zomorodian N, et al. Phase II study of pomegranate juice for men with rising prostate-specific antigen following surgery or radiation for prostate cancer. *Clin Cancer Res.* 2006;12(13):4018-26. http://www.ncbi.nlm.nih.gov.
723. Malik A, Mukhtar H. Prostate cancer prevention through pomegranate fruit. *Cell Cycle.* 2006;5(4):371-3. http://www.ncbi.nlm.nih.gov.
724. Malik A, Afaq F, Sarfaraz S, Adhami VM, Syed DN, Mukhtar H. Pomegranate fruit juice for chemoprevention and chemotherapy of prostate cancer. *Proc Natl Acad Sci U S A.* 200511;102(41):14813-8. http://www.ncbi.nlm.nih.gov.
725. Faria A, Calhau C. The bioactivity of pomegranate: impact on health and disease. *Crit Rev Food Sci Nutr.* 2011;51(7):626-34. http://www.ncbi.nlm.nih.gov.
726. Li Q, Kakizaki M, Sugawara Y, Tomata Y, Watanabe T, Nishino Y, Tsuji I. Coffee consumption and the risk of prostate cancer: the Ohsaki Cohort Study. *Br J Cancer.* 2013;108(11):2381-9. http://www.ncbi.nlm.nih.gov.
727. Discacciati A, Orsini N, Andersson SO, Andrén O, Johansson JE, Mantzoros CS, Wolk A. Coffee consumption and risk of localized, advanced and fatal prostate cancer: a population-based prospective study. *Ann Oncol.* 2013;24(7):1912-8. http://www.ncbi.nlm.nih.gov.
728. Yu X, Bao Z, Zou J, Dong J. Coffee consumption and risk of cancers: a meta-analysis of cohort studies. *BMC Cancer.* 2011;11:96. http://www.ncbi.nlm.nih.gov.

729. Shafique K, McLoone P, Qureshi K, Leung H, Hart C, Morrison DS. Coffee consumption and prostate cancer risk: further evidence for inverse relationship. *Nutr J.* 2012;11:42. http://www.ncbi.nlm.nih.gov.

730. Wilson KM, Kasperzyk JL, Rider JR, Kenfield S, van Dam RM, Stampfer MJ, Giovannucci E, Mucci LA. Coffee consumption and prostate cancer risk and progression in the Health Professionals Follow-up Study. *J Natl Cancer Inst.* 2011;103(11):876-84. http://www.ncbi.nlm.nih.gov.

731. Food, Nutrition, Physical Activity, and the Prevention of Cancer a Global Perspective. World Cancer Research Fund/American Institute for Cancer Research; 2007.

732. Chan DS, Lau R, Aune D, Vieira R, Greenwood DC, Kampman E, Norat T. Red and Processed Meat and Colorectal Cancer Incidence: Meta-Analysis of Prospective Studies. *PLoS One.* 2011;6(6):e20456. http://www.ncbi.nlm.nih.gov.

733. Johnson CM, Wei C, Ensor JE, Smolenski DJ, Amos CI, Levin B, Berry DA. Meta-analyses of colorectal cancer risk factors. *Cancer Causes Control.* 2013;24(6):1207-22.

734. Chao A, Thun MJ, Connell CJ, et al. Meat consumption and risk of colorectal cancer. *JAMA.* 2005;293(2):172-82. http://www.ncbi.nlm.nih.gov.

735. Le Marchand L, Hankin JH, Pierce LM, et al. Well-done red meat, metabolic phenotypes and colorectal cancer in Hawaii. *Mutat Res.* 2002;506-507:205-14. http://www.ncbi.nlm.nih.gov.

736. Food, Nutrition, Physical Activity, and the Prevention of Cancer: a Global Perspective. World Cancer Research Fund/American Institute for Cancer Research; 2007. http://www.dietandcancerreport.org

737. Mai V, McCrary QM, Sinha R, Glei M. Associations between dietary habits and body mass index with gut microbiota composition and fecal water genotoxicity: an observational study in African American and Caucasian American volunteers. Nutr J. 2009;8:49. http://www.ncbi.nlm.nih.gov.

738. Garland CF, et al. Do sunlight and vitamin D reduce the likelihood of colon cancer? *Int. J. Epidemiol.* 1980;9:227–231. http://www.ncbi.nlm.nih.gov.

739. McCullough ML, et al. Calcium, vitamin D, dairy products, and risk of colorectal cancer in the Cancer Prevention Study II Nutrition Cohort (United States) . *Cancer Causes Control.* 2003;14:1–12. http://www.ncbi.nlm.nih.gov.

740. Lieberman DA, et al. Risk factors for advanced colonic neoplasia and hyp. erplastic polyps in asymptomatic individuals. . *JAMA.* 2003;290:2959–2967. http://www.ncbi.nlm.nih.gov.

741. Freedman DM, et al. Prospective study of serum vitamin D and cancer mortality in the United States. . *J. Natl Cancer Inst.* 2007;99:1594–1602.

http://www.ncbi.nlm.nih.gov.

742. Larsson SC, Bergkvist L, Wolk A. Consumption of sugar and sugar-sweetened foods and the risk of pancreatic cancer in a prospective study. *Am J Clin Nutr.* 2006;84(5):1171-6. http://www.ncbi.nlm.nih.gov.

743. Chan JM, Wang F, Holly EA. Sweets, sweetened beverages, and risk of pancreatic cancer in a large population-based case-control study. *Cancer Causes Control.* 2009;20(6):835-46. http://www.ncbi.nlm.nih.gov.

744. Schernhammer ES, Hu FB, Giovannucci E, Michaud DS, Colditz GA, Stampfer MJ, Fuchs CS. Sugar-sweetened soft drink consumption and risk of pancreatic cancer in two prospective cohorts. *Cancer Epidemiol Biomarkers Prev.* 2005;14(9):2098-105. http://www.ncbi.nlm.nih.gov.

745. Genkinger JM, Li R, Spiegelman D, et al. Coffee, tea, and sugar-sweetened carbonated soft drink intake and pancreatic cancer risk: a pooled analysis of 14 cohort studies. *Cancer Epidemiol Biomarkers Prev.* 2012;21(2):305-18. http://www.ncbi.nlm.nih.gov.

746. Mueller NT, Odegaard A, Anderson K, Yuan JM, Gross M, Koh WP, Pereira MA. Soft drink and juice consumption and risk of pancreatic cancer: the Singapore Chinese Health Study. *Cancer Epidemiol Biomarkers Prev.* 2010;19(2):447-55. http://www.ncbi.nlm.nih.gov.

747. Michaud DS, Liu S, Giovannucci E, Willett WC, Colditz GA, Fuchs CS. Dietary sugar, glycemic load, and pancreatic cancer risk in a prospective study. *J Natl Cancer Inst.* 2002;94(17):1293-300. http://www.ncbi.nlm.nih.gov.

748. Schernhammer ES, Hu FB, Giovannucci E, Michaud DS, Colditz GA, Stampfer MJ, Fuchs CS. Sugar-sweetened soft drink consumption and risk of pancreatic cancer in two prospective cohorts. *Cancer Epidemiol Biomarkers Prev.* 2005;14(9):2098-105. http://www.ncbi.nlm.nih.gov.

749. Food, Nutrition, Physical Activity, and the Prevention of Cancer: a Global Perspective. Research. World Cancer Research Fund/American Institute for Cancer; 2007.

750. Food, Nutrition, Physical Activity, and the Prevention of Cancer: a Global Perspective. Research. World Cancer Research Fund/American Institute for Cancer; 2007.

751. Nutrition, Physical Activity, and the Prevention of Cancer: a Global Perspective. Research, World Cancer Research fund/American Institute for Cancer. Food; 2007.

752. Takata Y, Xiang YB, Yang G, Li H, Gao J, Cai H, Gao YT, Zheng W, Shu XO. Intakes of fruits, vegetables, and related vitamins and lung cancer risk:

results from the Shanghai Men's Health Study (2002-2009). *Nutr Cancer.* 2013;65(1):51-61. http://www.ncbi.nlm.nih.gov.

753. Dietary Supplement Fact Sheet: Vitamin B6. Bethesda, MD: Office of Dietary Supplements. National Institutes of Health; 2011.http://www.ods.od.nih.gov.

754. Dy GK, Bekele L, Hanson LJ, et al. Complementary and alternative medicine use by patients enrolled onto phase I clinical trials. J Clin Oncol. 2004 Dec 1;22(23):4810-5.

755. Richardson MA, Sanders T, Palmer JL, et al: Complementary/alternative medicine use in a comprehensive cancer center and the implications for oncology. J Clin Oncol 18:2505–2514, 2000

756. Zeeb H. Zellbiologie M, Greinert R. The Role of Vitamin D in Cancer Prevention (Does UV Protection Conflict With the Need to Raise Low Levels of Vitamin D?). *Dtsch Arztebl Int.* 2010; 107(37): 638–643. http://www.ncbi.nlm.nih.gov.

757. Garland CF, Garland FC, Gorham ED, Lipkin M, Newmark H, Mohr SB, Holick MF. The role of vitamin D in cancer prevention. *Am J Public Health.* 2006;96(2):252-61. http://www.ncbi.nlm.nih.gov.

758. Janowsky EC, Lester GE, Weinberg CR, et al. Association between low levels of 1,25-dihydroxyvitamin D and breast cancer risk. *Public Health Nutr.* 1999;2(3):283–291. http://www.ncbi.nlm.nih.gov.

759. Yao S, Zirpol Gi, Bovbjerg DH, Jandorf L, et al. Variants in the vitamin D pathway, serum levels of vitamin D, and estrogen receptor negative breast cancer among African-American women: a case-control study. *Breast Cancer Res.* 2012; 14(2): R58. http://www.ncbi.nlm.nih.gov.

760. Ahonen MH, Tenkanen L, Teppo L, Hakama M, Tuohimaa P. Prostate cancer risk and prediagnostic serum 25-hydroxyvitamin D levels (Finland). *Cancer Causes Control.* 2000;11(9): 847–852. http://www.ncbi.nlm.nih.gov.

761. Nesby-O'Dell S, Scanlon KS, Cogswell ME, et al. Hypovitaminosis D prevalence and determinants among African American and white women of reproductive age: third National Health and Nutrition Examination Survey, 1988–1994. *Am J Clin Nutr.* 2002; 76(1):187–192. http://www.ncbi.nlm.nih.gov.

762. Awamey E, Hollis B, Bell N. Low serum 25-hydroxyvitamin D in blacks results from decreased production rate and not increased metabolic clearance rate . *J Bone Miner Res.* 1996; 11:S165. http://www.ncbi.nlm.nih.gov.

763. Clemens TL, Adams JS, Henderson SL, Holick MF. Increased skin pigment reduces the capacity of skin to synthesise vitamin D3. *Lancet.* 1982;1(8263):74-6. http://www.ncbi.nlm.nih.gov.

764. Matsuoka LY, Ide L, Wortsman J, MacLaughlin JA, Holick MF. Sunscreens suppress cutaneous vitamin D3 synthesis. *J Clin Endocrinol Metab.* 1987;64(6):1165-8. http://www.ncbi.nlm.nih.gov.

765. Matsuoka LY, Wortsman J, Hanifan N, Holick MF. Chronic sunscreen use decreases circulating concentrations of 25-hydroxyvitamin D. A preliminary study. *Arch Dermatol.* 1988;124(12):1802-4. http://www.ncbi.nlm.nih.gov.

766. Garland CF, Garland FC, Gorham ED, et al. The Role of Vitamin D in Cancer Prevention. *Am J Public Health.* 2006; 96(2): 252–261. http://www.ncbi.nlm.nih.gov.

767. Nakamura K, Nashimoto M, Hori Y, Yamamoto M. Serum 25-hydroxyvitamin D concentrations and related dietary factors in peri- and postmenopausal Japanese women. *Am J Clin Nutr.* 2000;71:1161–1165. http://www.ncbi.nlm.nih.gov.

768. Brasky TM, Lampe JW, Potte JDr, Patterson RE, White E. Specialty Supplements and Breast Cancer Risk in the VITamins And Lifestyle (VITAL) Cohort. *Cancer Epidemiol Biomarkers Prev.* 2010;19(7):1696-708. http://www.ncbi.nlm.nih.gov.

769. Mandal CC, Triparna Ghosh-Choudhury T, Yoneda T, et al. Fish oil prevents breast cancer cell metastasis to bone. *Biochem Biophys Res Commun.* 2010; 402(4): 602–607. http://www.ncbi.nlm.nih.gov.

770. Torfadottir JE, Valdimarsdottir UA, Mucci LA, et al. Consumption of Fish Products across the Lifespan and Prostate Cancer Risk. *PLoS One.* 2013; 8(4): e59799. http://www.ncbi.nlm.nih.gov.

771. Murphy RA, Mourtzakis M, Chu QS, Baracos VE, Reiman T, Mazurak VC. Supplementation with fish oil increases first-line chemotherapy efficacy in patients with advanced nonsmall cell lung cancer. *Cancer.* 2011;117(16):3774-80. http://www.ncbi.nlm.nih.gov.

772. Yam D, Peled A, Shinitzky M. Suppression of tumor growth and metastasis by dietary fish oil combined with vitamins E and C and cisplatin. *Cancer Chemother Pharmacol.* 2001;47(1):34-40. http://www.ncbi.nlm.nih.gov.

773. Bonatto SJ, Oliveira HH, Nunes EA, et al. Fish oil supplementation improves neutrophil function during cancer chemotherapy. *Lipids.* 2012;47(4):383-9. http://www.ncbi.nlm.nih.gov.

774. Chen J, Stavro PM, Thompson LU. Dietary flaxseed inhibits human breast cancer growth and metastasis and downregulates expression of insulin-like growth factor and epidermal growth factor receptor. *Nutr Cancer.* 2002;43(2):187-92. http://www.ncbi.nlm.nih.gov.

775. Bergman Jungeström M, Thompson LU, Dabrosin C. Flaxseed and its lignans inhibit estradiol-induced growth, angiogenesis, and secretion of vascular endothelial growth factor in human breast cancer xenografts in vivo. *Clin Cancer Res.* 20071;13(3):1061-7. http://www.ncbi.nlm.nih.gov.

776. Chen J, Wang L, Thompson LU. Flaxseed and its components reduce metastasis after surgical excision of solid human breast tumor in nude mice. *Cancer Lett.* 2006;234(2):168-75. http://www.ncbi.nlm.nih.gov.

777. Saggar JK, Chen J, Corey P, Thompson LU. Dietary flaxseed lignan or oil combined with tamoxifen treatment affects MCF-7 tumor growth through estrogen receptor- and growth factor-signaling pathways. *Mol Nutr Food Res.* 2010;54(3):415-25. http://www.ncbi.nlm.nih.gov.

778. Demark-Wahnefried W, Polascik TJ, George SL, et al. Flaxseed supplementation (not dietary fat restriction) reduces prostate cancer proliferation rates in men presurgery. *Cancer Epidemiol Biomarkers Prev.* 2008;17(12):3577-87. http://www.ncbi.nlm.nih.gov.

779. Lin X, Gingrich JR, Bao W, Li J, Haroon ZA, Demark-Wahnefried W. Effect of flaxseed supplementation on prostatic carcinoma in transgenic mice.. *Urology.* 2002;60(5):919-24. http://www.ncbi.nlm.nih.gov.

780. Moragoda L, Jaszewski R, Majumdar APN. Curcumin induced modulation of cell cycle and apoptosis in gastric and colon cancer cells, Anticancer Research. 2001;21(2):873–878. http://www.ncbi.nlm.nih.gov.

781. Azuine MA, Bhide SV. Chemopreventive effect of turmeric against stomach and skin tumors induced by chemical carcinogens in Swiss mice. Nutrition and Cancer, 1992; 17(1):77–83. http://www.ncbi.nlm.nih.gov.

782. Dorai T, Cao YC, Dorai B, Buttyan R, Katz AE. Therapeutic potential of curcumin in human prostate cancer. III. Curcumin inhibits proliferation, induces apoptosis, and inhibits angiogenesis of LNCaP prostate cancer cells in vivo. Prostate. 2001;47(4):293–303. http://www.ncbi.nlm.nih.gov.

783. Lin SS, Lai KC, Hsu SC, et al. Curcumin inhibits the migration and invasion of human A549 lung cancer cells through the inhibition of matrix metalloproteinase- 2 and -9 and Vascular Endothelial Growth Factor (VEGF). *Cancer Lett.* 2009;285(2):127-33. http://www.ncbi.nlm.nih.gov.

784. Pelucchi C, Talamini R, Negri E, Levi F, Conti E, Franceschi S, La Vecchia C. Folate intake and risk of oral and pharyngeal cancer. *Ann Oncol.* 2003;14(11):1677-81. http://www.ncbi.nlm.nih.gov.

785. Rohan TE, Jain MG, Howe GR, Miller AB. Dietary folate consumption and breast cancer risk. *J Natl Cancer Inst.* 2000;92(3):266-9. http://www.ncbi.nlm.nih.gov.

786. Zhang S, Hunter DJ, Hankinson SE, Giovannucci EL, Rosner BA, Colditz GA, Speizer FE, Willett WC. A prospective study of folate intake and the risk of breast cancer. *JAMA.* 1999;281(17):1632-7. http://www.ncbi.nlm.nih.gov.

787. Zhang SM, Hankinson SE, Hunter DJ, Giovannucci EL, Colditz GA, Willett WC. Folate intake and risk of breast cancer characterized by hormone receptor status. *Cancer Epidemiol Biomarkers Prev.* 2005;14(8):2004-8. http://www.ncbi.nlm.nih.gov.

788. Sellers TA, Vierkant RA, Cerhan JR, et al. Interaction of dietary folate intake, alcohol, and risk of hormone receptor-defined breast cancer in a prospective study of postmenopausal women. *Cancer Epidemiol Biomarkers Prev.* 2002;11(10 Pt 1):1104-7. http://www.ncbi.nlm.nih.gov.

789. Hillman RS, Steinberg SE. The effects of alcohol on folate metabolism. *Annu Rev* Med.1982;33:345-354. http://www.ncbi.nlm.nih.gov.

790. Gaurav K, Goel RK, Shukla M, Pandey M. Glutamine: A novel approach to chemotherapy-induced toxicity. *J Med Paediatr Oncol.* 2012;33(1):13-20. http://www.ncbi.nlm.nih.gov.

791. Skubitz KM, Anderson PM. Oral glutamine to prevent chemotherapy induced stomatitis: a pilot study. *J Lab Clin Med.* 1996;127(2):223-8. http://www.ncbi.nlm.nih.gov.

792. Anderson PM, Schroeder G, Skubitz KM. Oral glutamine reduces the duration and severity of stomatitis after cytotoxic cancer chemotherapy. *Cancer.* 1998;83(7):1433-9. http://www.ncbi.nlm.nih.gov.

793. Vahdat L, Kyriakos P, Lange D, et al. Reduction of paclitaxel-induced peripheral neuropathy with glutamine. *Clin Cancer Res.* 2001;7:1192-1197. http://www.ncbi.nlm.nih.gov.

794. Wang WS, Lin JK, Lin TC, et al. Oral glutamine is effective for preventing oxaliplatin-induced neuropathy in colorectal cancer patients. *Oncologist.* 2007;12(3):312-9.http://www.ncbi.nlm.nih.gov.

795. Stubblefield MD, Vahdat LT, Balmaceda CM, et al. Glutamine as a neuroprotective agent in high-dose paclitaxel-induced peripheral neuropathy: a clinical and electrophysiologic study. *Clin Oncol (R Coll Radiol).* 2005;17(4):271-6. http://www.ncbi.nlm.nih.gov.

796. Song XD, Zhang JJ, Wang MR, Liu WB, Gu XB, Lv CJ. Astaxanthin induces mitochondria-mediated apoptosis in rat hepatocellular carcinoma CBRH-7919 cells. *Biol Pharm Bull.* 2011;34(6):839-44. http://www.ncbi.nlm.nih.gov.

797. Yasui Y, Hosokawa M, Mikami N, Miyashita K, Tanaka T. Dietary astaxanthin inhibits colitis and colitis-associated colon carcinogenesis in mice via modulation of the inflammatory cytokines. *Chem Biol Interact.* 2011;193(1):79-87. http://www.ncbi.nlm.nih.gov.

798. Nagendraprabhu P, Sudhandiran G. Astaxanthin inhibits tumor invasion by decreasing extracellular matrix production and induces apoptosis in experimental rat colon carcinogenesis by modulating the expressions of ERK-2, NFkB and COX-2. *Invest New Drugs.* 2011;29(2):207-24.

799. Nakao R, Nelson OL, Park JS, Mathison BD, Thompson PA, Chew BP. Effect of dietary astaxanthin at different stages of mammary tumor initiation in BALB/c mice. *Anticancer Res.* 2010;30(6):2171-5. http://www.ncbi.nlm.nih.gov.

800. Jyonouchi H, Sun S, Iijima K, Gross MD. Antitumor activity of astaxanthin and its mode of action. *Nutr Cancer.* 2000;36(1):59-65. http://www.ncbi.nlm.nih.gov.

801. Chew BP, Park JS, Wong MW, Wong TS. A comparison of the anticancer activities of dietary beta-carotene, canthaxanthin and astaxanthin in mice in vivo. *Anticancer Res.* 1999;19(3A):1849-53. http://www.ncbi.nlm.nih.gov.

802. Prabhu PN, Ashokkumar P, Sudhandiran G. Antioxidative and antiproliferative effects of astaxanthin during the initiation stages of 1,2-dimethyl hydrazine-induced experimental colon carcinogenesis. *Fundam Clin Pharmacol.* 2009;23(2):225-34. http://www.ncbi.nlm.nih.gov.

803. Tanaka T, Morishita Y, Suzui M, Kojima T, Okumura A, Mori H. Chemoprevention of mouse urinary bladder carcinogenesis by the naturally occurring carotenoid astaxanthin. *Carcinogenesis.* 1994;15(1):15-9. http://www.ncbi.nlm.nih.gov.

804. Kurihara H, Koda H, Asami S, Kiso Y, Tanaka T. Contribution of the antioxidative property of astaxanthin to its protective effect on the promotion of cancer metastasis in mice treated with restraint stress. *Life Sci.* 2002;70(21):2509-20. http://www.ncbi.nlm.nih.gov.

805. Anderson ML. A preliminary investigation of the enzymatic inhibition of 5alpha-reduction and growth of prostatic carcinoma cell line LNCap-FGC by natural astaxanthin and Saw Palmetto lipid extract in vitro. *J Herb Pharmacother.* 2005;5(1):17-26. http://www.ncbi.nlm.nih.gov.

806. McCulloch M, See C, Shu XJ, et al. Astragalus-based Chinese herbs and platinum-based chemotherapy for advanced non-small-cell lung cancer: meta-analysis of randomized trials. *J Clin Oncol.* 2006;24(3):419-30. http://www.ncbi.nlm.nih.gov.

807. Shu X, McCulloch M, Xiao H, Broffman M, Gao J. Chinese herbal medicine and chemotherapy in the treatment of hepatocellular carcinoma: a meta-analysis of randomized controlled trials. *Integr Cancer Ther.* 2005;4(3):219-29. http://www.ncbi.nlm.nih.gov.

808. Robbins D, Gu X, Shi R, Liu J, Wang F, Ponville J, McCord JM, Zhao Y. The chemopreventive effects of Protandim: modulation of p53 mitochondrial translocation and apoptosis during skin carcinogenesis. *PLoS One.* 2010;5(7):e11902. http://www.ncbi.nlm.nih.gov.

809. Liu J, Gu X, Robbins D, Li G, Shi R, McCord JM, Zhao Y. Protandim, a fundamentally new antioxidant approach in chemoprevention using mouse two-stage skin carcinogenesis as a model. *PLoS One.* 2009;4(4):e5284. http://www.ncbi.nlm.nih.gov.

810. Tröger W, Zdrale Z, Stanković N, Matijašević M. Five-Year Follow-Up of Patients with Early Stage Breast Cancer After a Randomized Study Comparing Additional Treatment with Viscum Album (L.) Extract to Chemotherapy Alone. *Breast Cancer (Auckl).* 2012;6:173-80. http://www.ncbi.nlm.nih.gov.

811. Kim KC, Yook JH, Eisenbraun J, Kim BS, Huber R. Quality of life, immunomodulation and safety of adjuvant mistletoe treatment in patients with gastric carcinoma - a randomized, controlled pilot study. *BMC Complement Altern Med.* 2012;12:172. http://www.ncbi.nlm.nih.gov.

812. Podlech O, Harter PN, Mittelbronn M, Pöschel S, Naumann U. Fermented mistletoe extract as a multimodal antitumoral agent in gliomas. *Evid Based Complement Alternat Med.* 2012;2012:501796. http://www.ncbi.nlm.nih.gov.

813. Uçar EÖ, Arda N, Aitken A. Extract from mistletoe, Viscum album L., reduces Hsp27 and 14-3-3 protein expression and induces apoptosis in C6 rat glioma cells. *Genet Mol Res.* 2012;11(3):2801-13. http://www.ncbi.nlm.nih.gov.

814. Lee JE, Lee RA, Kim KH, Lee JH. Induction of apoptosis with diallyl disulfide in AGS gastric cancer cell line. *J Korean Surg Soc.* 2011;81(2):85-95. http://www.ncbi.nlm.nih.gov.

815. Wang X, Jiao F, Wang QW, et al. Aged black garlic extract induces inhibition of gastric cancer cell growth in vitro and in vivo. *Mol Med Rep.* 2012;5(1):66-72. http://www.ncbi.nlm.nih.gov.

816. Hirsch K, Danilenko M, Giat J, et al. Effect of purified allicin, the major ingredient of freshly crushed garlic, on cancer cell proliferation. *Nutr Cancer.* 2000;38(2):245-54. http://www.ncbi.nlm.nih.gov.

817. Bat-Chen W, Golan T, Peri I, Ludmer Z, Schwartz B. Allicin purified from fresh garlic cloves induces apoptosis in colon cancer cells via Nrf2. *Nutr Cancer.* 2010;62(7):947-57. http://www.ncbi.nlm.nih.gov.

818. Liu Z, Li M, Chen K, et al. S-allylcysteine induces cell cycle arrest and apoptosis in androgen-independent human prostate cancer cells. *Mol Med Rep.* 2012;5(2):439-43. http://www.ncbi.nlm.nih.gov.

819. Pei Y, Wu B, Cao Q, Wu L, Yang G. Hydrogen sulfide mediates the anti-survival effect of sulforaphane on human prostate cancer cells. *Toxicol Appl Pharmacol.* 2011;257(3):420-8. http://www.ncbi.nlm.nih.gov.

820. Pai MH, Kuo YH, Chiang EP, Tang FY. S-Allylcysteine inhibits tumour progression and the epithelial-mesenchymal transition in a mouse xenograft model of oral cancer. *Br J Nutr.* 2012;108(1):28-38. http://www.ncbi.nlm.nih.gov.

821. Tsubura A, Lai YC, Kuwata M, Uehara N, Yoshizawa K. Anticancer effects of garlic and garlic-derived compounds for breast cancer control. *Anticancer Agents Med Chem.* 2011;11(3):249-53. http://www.ncbi.nlm.nih.gov.

822. Nakagawa H, Tsuta K, Kiuchi K, et al. Growth inhibitory effects of diallyl disulfide on human breast cancer cell lines. *Carcinogenesis.* 2001;22(6):891-7. http://www.ncbi.nlm.nih.gov.

823. Brasky TM, Kristal AR, Navarro SL, Lampe JW, Peters U, Patterson RE, White E. Specialty supplements and prostate cancer risk in the VITamins and Lifestyle (VITAL) cohort. *Nutr Cancer.* 2011;63(4):573-82. http://www.ncbi.nlm.nih.gov.

824. Raina K, Singh RP, Agarwal R, Agarwal C. Oral grape seed extract inhibits prostate tumor growth and progression in TRAMP mice. *Cancer Res.* 2007;67(12):5976-82. http://www.ncbi.nlm.nih.gov.

825. Vayalil PK, Mittal A, Katiyar SK. Proanthocyanidins from grape seeds inhibit expression of matrix metalloproteinases in human prostate carcinoma cells, which is associated with the inhibition of activation of MAPK and NF kappa B. *Carcinogenesis.* 2004;25(6):987-95. http://www.ncbi.nlm.nih.gov.

825. Jang M, Cai L, Udeani GO, et al. Cancer chemopreventive activity of resveratrol, a natural product derived from grapes. *Science.* 1997;275(5297):218-20. http://www.ncbi.nlm.nih.gov.

827. Tyagi A, Agarwal R, Agarwal C. Grape seed extract inhibits EGF-induced a nd constitutively active mitogenic signaling but activates JNK in human prostate carcinoma DU145 cells: possible role in antiproliferation and apoptosis. *Oncogene.* 2003;22(9):1302-16. http://www.ncbi.nlm.nih.gov.

828. Agarwal C, Tyagi A, Agarwal R. Gallic acid causes inactivating phosphorylation of cdc25A/cdc25C-cdc2 via ATM-Chk2 activation, leading to cell cycle arrest, and induces apoptosis in human prostate carcinoma DU145 cells. *Mol Cancer Ther.* 2006(12):3294-302. http://www.ncbi.nlm.nih.gov.

829. Veluri R, Singh RP, Liu Z, Thompson JA, Agarwal R, Agarwal C. Fractionation of grape seed extract and identification of gallic acid as one of the major active constituents causing growth inhibition and apoptotic death of DU145 human prostate carcinoma cells. *Carcinogenesis.* 2006;27(7):1445-53. http://www.ncbi.nlm.nih.gov.

830. Jankun J, Selman SH, Swiercz R, Skrzypczak-Jankun E. Why drinking green tea could prevent cancer. *Nature.* 1997;387(6633):561. http://www.ncbi.nlm.nih.gov.

831. de Pace RC, Liu X, Sun M, et al. Anticancer activities of (-)-epigallocatechin-3-gallate encapsulated nanoliposomes in MCF7 breast cancer cells. *J Liposome Res.* 2013;23(3):187-96. http://www.ncbi.nlm.nih.gov.

832. Thangapazham RL, Passi N, Maheshwari RK. Green tea polyphenol and epigallocatechin gallate induce apoptosis and inhibit invasion in human breast cancer cells. *Cancer Biol Ther.* 2007;6(12):1938-43. http://www.ncbi.nlm.nih.gov.

833. Dou QP, Landis-Piwowar KR, Chen D, Huo C, Wan SB, Chan TH. Green tea polyphenols as a natural tumour cell proteasome inhibitor. *Inflammopharmacology.* 2008;16(5):208-12. http://www.ncbi.nlm.nih.gov.

834. Fujiki H. Two stages of cancer prevention with green tea. *J Cancer Res Clin Oncol.* 1999;125(11):589-97. http://www.ncbi.nlm.nih.gov.

835. Popiela T, Kulig J, Hanisch J, Bock PR. Influence of a complementary treatment with oral enzymes on patients with colorectal cancers--an epidemiological retrolective cohort study. *Cancer Chemother Pharmacol.* 2001;47 Suppl:S55-63. http://www.ncbi.nlm.nih.gov.

836. Beuth J, Ost B, Pakdaman A, et al. Impact of complementary oral enzyme application on the postoperative treatment results of breast cancer patients--results of an epidemiological multicentre retrolective cohort study. *Cancer Chemother Pharmacol.* 2001;47 Suppl:S45-54.

837. Sakalová A, Bock PR, Dedík L, et al. Retrolective cohort study of an additive therapy with an oral enzyme preparation in patients with multiple myeloma. *Cancer Chemother Pharmacol.* 2001;47 Suppl:S38-44. http://www.ncbi.nlm.nih.gov.

838. Osterlund P, Ruotsalainen T, Korpela R, et al. Lactobacillus supplementation for diarrhoea related to chemotherapy of colorectal cancer: a randomised study. *Br J Cancer.* 2007;97(8):1028-34. http://www.ncbi.nlm.nih.gov.

839. Salminen E, Elomaa I, Minkkinen J, Vapaatalo H, Salminen S. Preservation of intestinal integrity during radiotherapy using live Lactobacillusacidophilus cultures. *Clin Radiol.* 1988;39:435–437.

840. Urbancsek H, Kazar T, Mezes I, Neumann K. Results of a double-blind, randomized study to evaluate the efficacy and safety of Antibiophilus in patients with radiation-induced diarrhoea. *Eur J Gastroenterol Hepatol.* 2001;13(4):391-6. http://www.ncbi.nlm.nih.gov.

841. Pommier P, Gomez F, Sunyach MP, D'Hombres A, Carrie C, Montbarbon X. Phase III randomized trial of Calendula officinalis compared with trolamine for the prevention of acute dermatitis during irradiation for breast cancer. *J Clin Oncol.* 2004;22(8):1447-53. http://www.ncbi.nlm.nih.gov.

842. Schlappack O. Homeopathic treatment of radiation-induced itching in breast cancer patients. A prospective observational study. *Homeopathy.* 2004;93(4):210-5. http://www.ncbi.nlm.nih.gov.

843. Thompson EA, Reilly D. The homeopathic approach to the treatment of symptoms of oestrogen withdrawal in breast cancer patients. A prospective observational study. *Homeopathy.* 2003;92(3):131-4. http://www.ncbi.nlm.nih.gov.

844. Oberbaum M, Yaniv I, Ben-Gal Y et al. A randomized, controlled clinical trial of the homeopathic medication TRAUMEEL S in the treatment of chemotherapy-induced stomatitis in children undergoing stem cell transplantation. *Cancer.* 2001;92(3):684-90.

845. Otte JL, Carpenter JS, Zhong X, Johnstone PA. Feasibility study of acupuncture for reducing sleep disturbances and hot flashes in postmenopausal breast cancer survivors. *Clin Nurse Spec.* 2011;25(5):228-36. http://www.ncbi.nlm.nih.gov.

846. Crew KD, Capodice JL, Greenlee H, et al. Pilot study of acupuncture for the treatment of joint symptoms related to adjuvant aromatase inhibitor therapy in postmenopausal breast cancer patients. *J Cancer Surviv.* 2007;1(4):283-91. http://www.ncbi.nlm.nih.gov.

847. Crew KD, Capodice JL, Greenlee H, et al. Randomized, blinded, sham-controlled trial of acupuncture for the management of aromatase inhibitor-associated joint symptoms in women with early-stage breast cancer. *J Clin Oncol.* 2010;28(7):1154-60. http://www.ncbi.nlm.nih.gov.

848. Cho JH, Chung WK, Kang W, et al. Manual acupuncture improved quality of life in cancer patients with radiation-induced xerostomia. *J Altern Complement Med.* 2008;14(5):523-6. 919.

849. Blom M, Dawidson I, Fernberg JO, Johnson G, Angmar-Månsson B. Acupuncture treatment of patients with radiation-induced xerostomia. *Eur J Cancer B Oral Oncol.* 1996;32B(3):182-90.

850. Wong RK, Jones GW, Sagar SM, Babjak AF, Whelan T. A Phase I-II study in the use of acupuncture-like transcutaneous nerve stimulation in the treatment of radiation-induced xerostomia in head-and-neck cancer patients treated with radical radiotherapy. *Int J Radiat Oncol Biol Phys.* 2003 1;57(2):472-80. http://www.ncbi.nlm.nih.gov.

851. Feng Y, Wang XY, Li SD, et al. Clinical research of acupuncture on malignant tumor patients for improving depression and sleep quality. *J Tradit Chin Med.* 2011;31(3):199-202. http://www.ncbi.nlm.nih.gov.

852. Donald GK, Tobin I, Stringer J. Evaluation of acupuncture in the management of chemotherapy-induced peripheral neuropathy. *Acupunct Med.* 2011;29(3):230-3. http://www.ncbi.nlm.nih.gov.

853. Schroeder S, Meyer-Hamme G, Epplée S. Acupuncture for chemotherapy-induced peripheral neuropathy (CIPN): a pilot study using neurography. *Acupunct Med.* 2012;30(1):4-7. http://www.ncbi.nlm.nih.gov.

854. Schröder S, Liepert J, Remppis A, Greten JH. Acupuncture treatment improves nerve conduction in peripheral neuropathy. *Eur J Neurol.* 2007;14(3):276-81. http://www.ncbi.nlm.nih.gov.

855. Wong R, Sagar S. Acupuncture treatment for chemotherapy-induced peripheral neuropathy--a case series. *Eur J Neurol.* 2007;14(3):276-81. http://www.ncbi.nlm.nih.gov.

856. Nystrom E, Ridderstrom G, Leffler AS. Manual acupuncture as an adjunctive treatment of nausea in patients with cancer in palliative care--a prospective, observational pilot study. Acupunct Med. 2008;26(1):27-32. http://www.ncbi.nlm.nih.gov.

857. Reindl TK, Geilen W, Hartmann R, et al. Acupuncture against chemotherapy-induced nausea and vomiting in pediatric oncology. Interim results of a multicenter crossover study. *Support Care Cancer.* 2006;14(2):172-6.

858. Hyperthermia in Cancer Treatment. Bethesda, MD, National Cancer Institute. National Institutes of Health. http:// www.cancer.gov.

859. van der Zee J. Heating the patient: a promising approach? Ann Oncol. 2002; 13(8):1173-84.

860. Wust P, Hildebrandt B, Sreenivasa G, et al. Hyperthermia in combined treatment of cancer. *Lancet Oncol.* 2002;3(8):487-97.

861. Falk MH, Issels RD. Hyperthermia in oncology. *Int J Hyperthermia.* 2001; 17(1):1-18. http://www.ncbi.nlm.nih.gov.

862. Manning MR, Cetas TC, Miller RC, Oleson JR, Connor WG, Gerner EW. Clinical hyperthermia: results of a phase I trial employing hyperthermia alone or in combination with external beam or interstitial radiotherapy. *Cancer.* 1982;49(2):205-16. http://www.ncbi.nlm.nih.gov.

863. van der Zee J. Heating the patient: a promising approach? *Ann Oncol.* 2002; 13(8):1173-84. http://www.ncbi.nlm.nih.gov.

864. Ferrell-Torry AT, Glick OJ. The use of therapeutic massage as a nursing intervention to modify anxiety and the perception of cancer pain. *Cancer Nurs.* 1993;16(2):93-101. http://www.ncbi.nlm.nih.gov.

865. Toth M, Marcantonio ER, Davis RB, et al. Massage Therapy for Patients with Metastatic Cancer: A Pilot Randomized Controlled Trial. *J Altern Complement Med.* 2013;19(7):650-6.

866. Hughes D, Ladas E, Rooney D, Kelly K. Massage therapy as a supportive care intervention for children with cancer. *Oncol Nurs Forum.* 2008;35(3):431-42. http://www.ncbi.nlm.nih.gov.

867. Rexilius SJ, Mundt C, Erickson Megel M, Agrawal S. Therapeutic effects of massage therapy and handling touch on caregivers of patients undergoing autologous hematopoietic stem cell transplant. *Oncol Nurs Forum.* 2002;29(3):E35-44. http://www.ncbi.nlm.nih.gov.

868. Wyatt G, Sikorskii A, Rahbar MH, Victorson D, You M. Health-related quality-of-life outcomes: a reflexology trial with patients with advanced-stage breast cancer. *Oncol Nurs Forum.* 2012;39(6):568-77. http://www.ncbi.nlm.nih.gov.

869. Stephenson NL, Weinrich SP, Tavakoli AS. The effects of foot reflexology on anxiety and pain in patients with breast and lung cancer. *Oncol Nurs Forum.* 2000;27(1):67-72. http://www.ncbi.nlm.nih.gov.

870. Stephenson NL, Swanson M, Dalton J, Keefe FJ, Engelke M. Partner-delivered reflexology: effects on cancer pain and anxiety. *Oncol Nurs Forum.* 2007; 34(1): 127-32. http://www.ncbi.nlm.nih.gov.

871. Buffart LM, van Uffelen JG, Riphagen II, et al. Physical and psychosocial benefits of yoga in cancer patients and survivors, a systematic review and meta-analysis of randomized controlled trials. *BMC Cancer.* 2012;12:559. http://www.ncbi.nlm.nih.gov.

872. Galantino ML, Greene L, Daniels L, Dooley B, Muscatello L, O'Donnell L. Longitudinal impact of yoga on chemotherapy-related cognitive impairment and quality of life in women with early stage breast cancer: a case series. *Explore (NY).* 2012;8(2):127-35. http://www.ncbi.nlm.nih.gov.

873. Dhruva A, Miaskowski C, Abrams D, et al. Yoga breathing for cancer chemotherapy-associated symptoms and quality of life: results of a pilot randomized controlled trial. *J Altern Complement Med.* 2012;18(5):473-9. http://www.ncbi.nlm.nih.gov.

874. Bruns F, et al. Selenium in the treatment of head and neck lymphedema. *Med Princ Pract.* 2004;13(4):185-90. http://www.ncbi.nlm.nih.gov.

875. Zimmermann T, Leonhardt H, Kersting S, Albrecht S, Range U, Eckelt U.Reduction of postoperative lymphedema after oral tumor surgery with sodium selenite. *Biol Trace Elem Res.* 2005;106(3):193-203. http://www.ncbi.nlm.nih.gov.

876. Kasseroller RG, Schrauzer GN. Treatment of secondary lymphedema of the arm with physical decongestive therapy and sodium selenite: a review. *Am J Ther.* 2000;7(4):273-9. http://www.ncbi.nlm.nih.gov.

877. Drews FA, Pasupathi M, Strayer DL. Passenger and cell phone conversations in simulated driving. *J Exp Psychol Appl.* 2008;14(4):392-400. http://www.ncbi.nlm.nih.gov.

878. Strayer DL, Johnston W A. Driven to distraction: Dual-task studies of simulated driving and conversing on a cellular phone. *Psychol Sci.* 2001;12(6):462-6. http://www.ncbi.nlm.nih.gov.

879. Strayer DL., Johnston W A. Driven to distraction: Dual-task studies of simulated driving and conversing on a cellular phone. *Psychol Sci.* 2001;12(6):462-6. http://www.ncbi.nlm.nih.gov.

880. Strayer DL, Drews FA. Profiles in driver distraction: effects of cell phone conversations on younger and older drivers. *Hum Factors.* 2004 Winter;46(4):640-9. http://www.ncbi.nlm.nih.gov.

881. Strayer DL, Drews FA. Cell-Phone-Induced Driver Distraction. Current Directions In Psychological Sicence. *Psychological Sicence.* 2007;16(3):128-131. http://www.ncbi.nlm.nih.gov.

882. Ishigami Y, Klein RM. Is a hands-free phone safer than a handheld phone? *J Safety Res.* 2009;40(2):157-64. http://www.ncbi.nlm.nih.gov.

883. Strayer DL, Drews FA, Johnston WA. Cell phone-induced failures of visual attention during simulated driving. *J Exp Psychol Appl.* 2003;9(1):23-32. http://www.ncbi.nlm.nih.gov.

884. Bicycle Helmet Use Laws. U.S. Department of Transportation. Washington, DC: National Highway Traffic Safety Administration; 2013. http://www.nhtsa.gov.

885. Blackman E. Helmet Protection against Traumatic Brain Injury: A Physics Perspective. University of Rochester. http://www.pas.rochester.edu.

886. U.S. dairy program subsidies. Washington, DC: Environmental Working Group; 2013. http://www.ewg.org.

887. Feskanich D, Willett WC, Stampfer MJ, Colditz GA. Milk, dietary calcium, and bone fractures in women: a 12-year prospective study. *Am J Public Health.* 1997;87(6):992-7. http://www.ncbi.nlm.nih.gov.

888. Owusu W, Willett WC, Feskanich D, Ascherio A, Spiegelman D, Colditz GA. Calcium intake and the incidence of forearm and hip fractures among men. *J Nutr.* 1997;127(9):1782-7. http://www.ncbi.nlm.nih.gov.

889. Wickham CA, Walsh K, Cooper C, et al. Dietary calcium, physical activity, and risk of hip fracture: a prospective study. *BMJ.* 1989; 299(6704): 889–892. http://www.ncbi.nlm.nih.gov.

890. Michaëlsson K, Holmberg L, Mallmin H, Sörensen S, Wolk A, Bergström R, Ljunghall S. Diet and hip fracture risk: a case-control study. Study Group of the Multiple Risk Survey on Swedish Women for Eating Assessment. *Int J Epidemiol.* 1995;24(4):771-82. http://www.ncbi.nlm.nih.gov.

891. Sampson H. Food allergy. *Journal of Allergy and Clinical Immunology.* 2003;111(2):540–547. http://www.ncbi.nlm.nih.gov.

892. Hip fracture incidence map. Switzerland: International Osteoporosis Foundation;2014.http://www.iofbonehealth.org.

893. Current Worldwide Total Milk Consumption per capita. ChartsBin;2007. http://chartsbin.com/view/1491.

894. Feskanich D, Willett WC, Colditz GA. Calcium, vitamin D, milk consumption, and hip fractures: a prospective study among postmenopausal women. *Am J Clin Nutr.* 2003;77(2):504-11.

895. Feskanich D, Weber P, Willett WC, Rockett H, Booth SL, Colditz GA. Vitamin K intake and hip fractures in women: a prospective study. *Am J Clin Nutr.* 1999;69(1):74-9. http://www.ncbi.nlm.nih.gov.

896. Booth SL, Tucker KL, Chen H, et al. Dietary vitamin K intakes are associated with hip fracture but not with bone mineral density in elderly men and women. *Am J Clin Nutr.* 2000;71(5):1201-8. http://www.ncbi.nlm.nih.gov.

897. Booth SL, Broe KE, Gagnon DR, et al. Vitamin K intake and bone mineral density in women and men. *Am J Clin Nutr.* 2003;77(2):512-6. http://www.ncbi.nlm.nih.gov.

898. Tucker KL, Hannan MT, Chen H, Cupples LA, Wilson PW, Kiel DP. Potassium, magnesium, and fruit and vegetable intakes are associated with greater bone mineral density in elderly men and women. *Am J Clin Nutr.* 1999;69(4):727-36. http://www.ncbi.nlm.nih.gov.

899. New SA, Bolton-Smith C, Grubb DA, Reid DM. Nutritional influences on bone mineral density: a cross sectional study of postmenopausal women. *Am J Clin Nutr.* 1997;65(6):1831-1839. http://www.ncbi.nlm.nih.gov.

900. Zhu K, Devine A, Prince RL. The effects of high potassium consumption on bone mineral density in a prospective cohort study of elderly postmenopausal women. *Osteoporos Int.* 2009;20(2):335-40. http://www.ncbi.nlm.nih.gov.

901. Feskanich D, Singh V, Willett WC, Colditz GA. Vitamin A intake and hip fractures among postmenopausal women. *JAMA.* 2002;287(1):47-54. http://www.ncbi.nlm.nih.gov.

902. Melhus H, Michaëlsson K, Kindmark A, et al. Excessive dietary intake of vitamin A is associated with reduced bone mineral density and increased risk for hip fracture. *Ann Intern Med.* 1998;129(10):770-8. http://www.ncbi.nlm.nih.gov.

903. Borer KT. Physical activity in the prevention and amelioration of osteoporosis in women : interaction of mechanical, hormonal and dietary factors. *Sports Med.* 2005;35(9):779-830. http://www.ncbi.nlm.nih.gov.

904. Lloyd T, Petit MA, Lin HM, Beck TJ. Lifestyle factors and the development of bone mass and bone strength in young women. *J Pediatr.* 2004;144(6):776-82. http://www.ncbi.nlm.nih.gov.

905. Lloyd T, Beck TJ, Lin HM, et al. Modifiable determinants of bone status in young women. *Bone.* 2002;30(2):416-21. http://www.ncbi.nlm.nih.gov.

906. Lloyd T, Chinchilli VM, Johnson-Rollings N, Kieselhorst K, Eggli DF, Marcus R. Adult female hip bone density reflects teenage sports-exercise patterns but not teenage calcium intake. *Pediatrics.* 2000;106(1 Pt 1):40-4. http://www.ncbi.nlm.nih.gov.

907. 2011 Bicycle and Pedestrian Fatalities, Mississippi Traffic Fatalities. Jackson, MS: MS Department of Public Safety; 2012. http://www.psdl.ssrc.msstate.edu.

908. Complete streets change travel patterns. Washington, DC: National Complete Street Coalition. http:// www.smartgrowthamerica.org.

909. National poll: Americans support funding for sidewalks and bikeways. America Bikes. 2012. http:// www.bikesbelong.org.

910. Manson JE, Greenland P, LaCroix AZ, et al. Walking compared with vigorous exercise for the prevention of cardiovascular events in women. *N Engl J Med.* 2002;347(10):716-25.

911. Manson J E, Hu F B, Rich, Edwards J W. et al. A prospective study of walking as compared with vigorous exercise in the prevention of coronary heart disease in women. *N Engl J Med* 1999. 341650–658.658.

912. Trivedi MH, Greer TL, Church TS, et al. Exercise as an augmentation treatment for nonremitted major depressive disorder: a randomized, parallel dose comparison. *J Clin Psychiatry.* 2011;72(5):677-84.

913. Middleton LE, Manini TM, Simonsick EM, et al. Activity energy expenditure and incident cognitive impairment in older adults. *Arch Intern Med.* 2011; 171(14):1251-7.

914. Yaffe K, Barnes D, Nevitt M, Lui LY, Covinsky K. A prospective study of physical activity and cognitive decline in elderly women: women who walk. *Arch Intern Med.* 2001;161(14):1703-8.

915. *Endurance exercise prevents premature aging.* Ontario, Canada:McMaster Univesity; 2011. http://fhs.mcmaster.ca/main/news/news_2011/exercise_and_aging_study.html

916. US National Library of Medicine. *Genetics Home Reference.* Bethesda, MD: National Institutes of Health.http://www.nlm.nih.gov.

917. Safdar A, Little JP, Stokl AJ, Hettinga BP, Akhtar M, Tarnopolsky MA. Exercise Increases Mitochondrial PGC-1α Content and Promotes Nuclear-Mitochondrial Cross-talk to Coordinate Mitochondrial Biogenesis. *J Biol Chem.* 2011; 286(12): 10605–10617.

918. *Interferon beta-1a Intramuscular Injection.* Bethesda, MD: American Society of Health-Systems Pharmacists, Inc. 2012. http://www.nlm.nih.gov.

919. World's Healthiest Foods. The George Mateljan Foundation. www.whfoods.com.

920. Yáñez JA, et al. Pharmacokinetics of selected chiral flavonoids: hesperetin, naringenin and eriodictyol in rats and their content in fruit juices. Biopharm Drug Dispos. 2008 Mar;29(2):63-82.

921. Koh E, Charoenprasert S, Mitchell AE. Effect of organic and conventional cropping systems on ascorbic acid, vitamin C, flavonoids, nitrate, and oxalate in 27 varieties of spinach (Spinacia oleracea L.). J Agric Food Chem. 2012 Mar 28;60(12):3144-50.

922. Mitchell AE, Hong YJ, Koh E, et al. Ten-year comparison of the influence of organic and conventional crop management practices on the content of flavonoids in tomatoes. J Agric Food Chem. 2007 Jul 25;55(15):6154-9.

923. Grinder-Pedersen L, Rasmussen SE, Bügel S, et al. Effect of diets based on foods from conventional versus organic production on intake and excretion of flavonoids and markers of antioxidative defense in humans. J Agric Food Chem. 2003;51(19):5671-6.

924. Asami DK, Hong YJ, Barrett DM, Mitchell AE. Comparison of the total phenolic and ascorbic acid content of freeze-dried and air-dried marionberry, strawberry, and corn grown using conventional, organic, and sustainable agricultural practices. J Agric Food Chem. 2003;51(5):1237-41.

925. Prior RL, Gu L, Wu X, et al. Plasma antioxidant capacity changes following a meal as a measure of the ability of a food to alter in vivo antioxidant status. *J Am Coll Nutr.* 2007;26(2):170-81.

926. Smith-Spangler C, Brandeau ML, Hunter GE, et al. Are organic foods safer or healthier than conventional alternatives?: a systematic review. *Ann Intern Med.* 2012;157(5):348-66.

927. Lu C, Toepel K, Irish R, Fenske RA, Barr DB, Bravo R. Organic diets significantly lower children's dietary exposure to organophosphorus pesticides. Environ Health Perspect. 2006;114(2):260-3.

928. The President's Cancer Panel. Reducing environmental cancer risk: What we can do now. Bethesda, MD: U.S. Health and Human Services; 2010. http://deainfo.nci.nih.gov.

929. Consumer demand drives growth in the organic food sector. Washington, DC. US Department of Agriculture.Economic Research Service;2013. http://www.ers.usda.gov.

930. USDA Organic Production and Handling Standards. Washington, DC. USDA National Organic Program;2011. http://www.ams.usda.gov.

931. The national list of allowed and prohibited substances: The national organic program. Washington, DC: USDA: 2014. http://www.ams.usda.gov.

Index

Author Bio

Getty Israel, MPH, is a dynamic public health practitioner who specializes in disease prevention and wellness through lifestyle change interventions. Also, she is an advocate for preventative-based public health policies.

> *"The most powerful therapy on the face of the Earth is not drug medications, dietary supplements, or invasive medical procedures; rather, it is a healthy lifestyle"*
>
> ~ Getty Israel

Made in the USA
Monee, IL
14 September 2026

63198305R00148